The Affordable Keto Diet Sweeties for Beginners

Quick, Easy and Delicious Keto Cakes and Bars

Jessica Simpson

I0135897

1

Contents

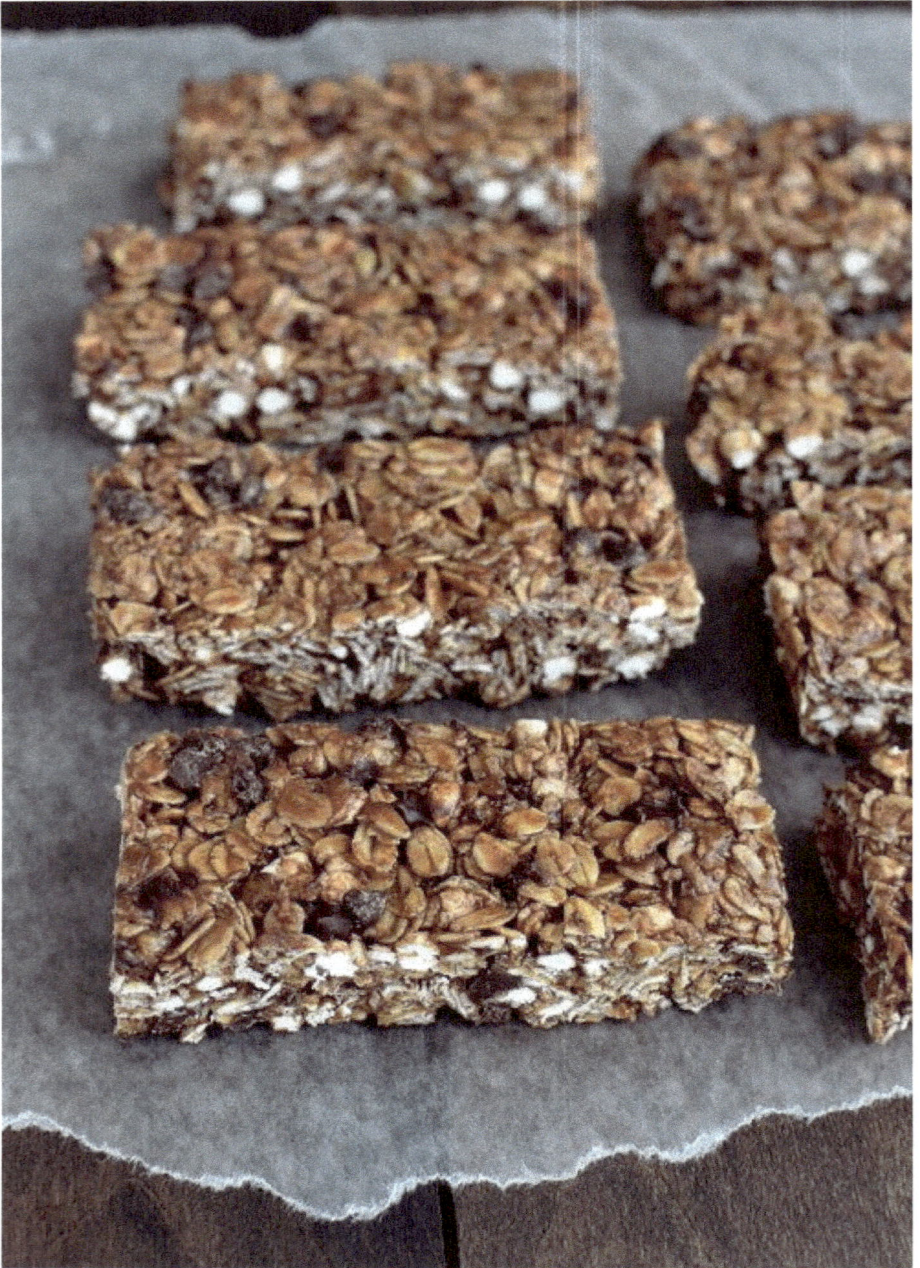

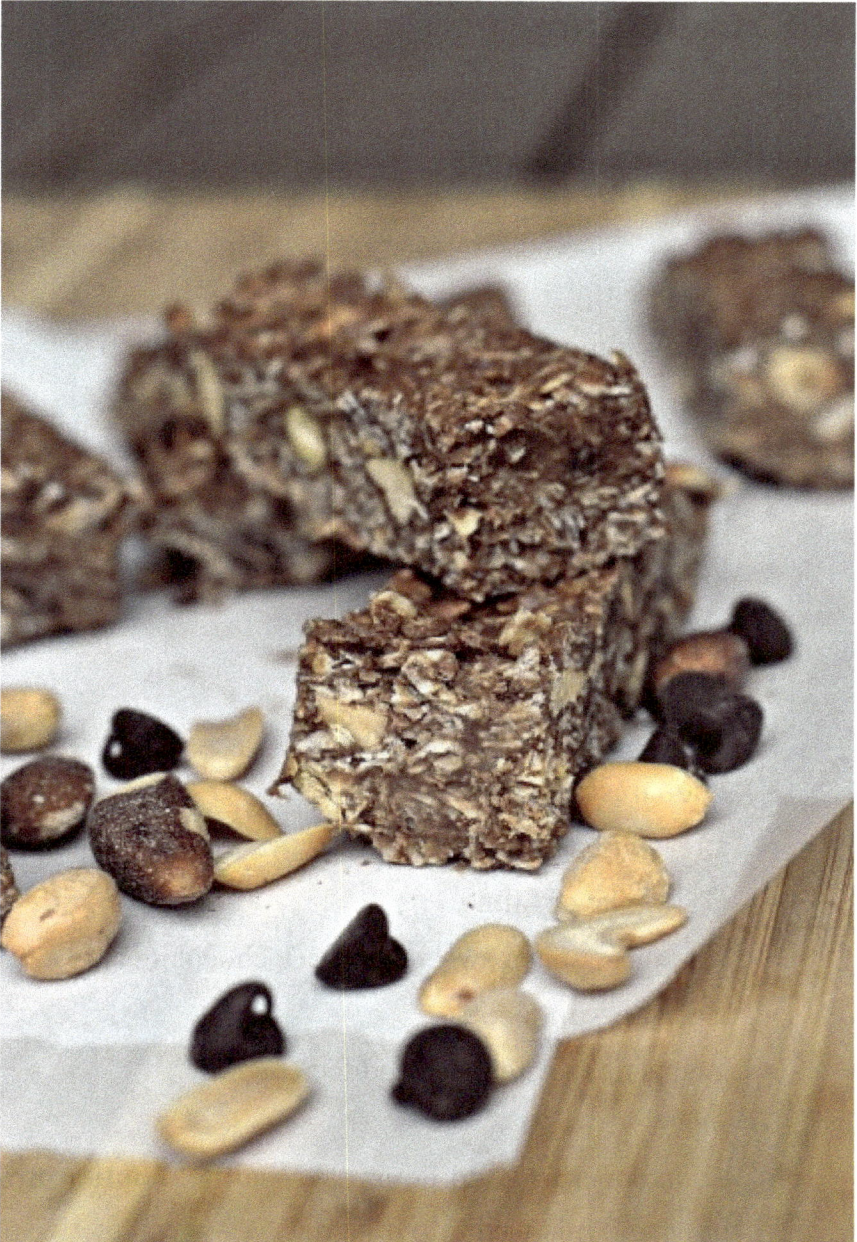

Keto Magic Bars

Servings: 24

Cooking Time: 30 Minutes

Ingredients:

- For crust:
- 2 cups almond flour
- 2 large eggs
- ½ teaspoon salt
- 4 tablespoons unsalted butter
- For condensed milk:
- 1 cup heavy cream
- 1 cup Swerve brown sugar
- 1/8 teaspoon salt
- 1 cup unsalted butter
- 2 teaspoons vanilla extract
- For top layer filling:
- 18 ounces stevia sweetened dark chocolate chips
- 2 cups pecan pieces
- 2 cups unsweetened shredded coconut

Directions:

1. To make crust: Add flour, eggs, salt and butter into a bowl and mix well into dough.

2. Transfer into a large, rectangular baking dish. Press the dough well onto the bottom of the dish. Pierce the dough at several places.

3. Bake in a preheated oven at 0° F for about 20-25 minutes or until light brown.

4. To make condensed milk: Add cream, Swerve, salt, butter and vanilla into a tall saucepan or pot.

5. When the milk mixture begins to boil, stir frequently for about 6 minutes or until thick like condensed milk. Turn off the heat and let it cool.

6. Scatter pecans, chocolate chips and coconut over the crust. Spoon the condensed milk over the crust.

7. Place the baking dish back in the oven and bake for 8 minutes.

8. Remove from the oven and cool for a while. Refrigerate for about an hour.

9. Slice into 24 bars and serve.

10. Leftovers can be stored in an airtight container in the refrigerator. These can keep for 4 – 5 days.

Nutrition Info: Per Servings: Calories: 395 kcal, Fat: 37.1 g, Carbohydrates: 5.8 g, Protein: 4 g

Chocolate Crunch Bars

Servings: 20

Cooking Time: 10 Minutes

Ingredients:

- 1 1/2 cups chocolate chips, stevia sweetened
- 1/2 cup monk fruit sweetener
- 1/4 cup coconut oil
- 1 cup almond butter
- 1 cup chopped almonds
- 1 cup chopped cashews
- 1 cup chopped pepitas

Directions:

1. Take an 8 by 8-inch baking dish, line with parchment paper and set aside until required.
2. Place chocolate chips in a heatproof bowl along with sweetener, oil and butter and microwave for 60 seconds or more until melted.
3. Stir well until combined, then stir in almonds, cashews, and pepitas and spread the mixture evenly into the baking dish.
4. Place the baking dish into the freezer for 1 hour or more until firm.

Nutrition Info: Calories: 1 Cal, Carbs: 4 g, Fat: 12 g, Protein: 7 g, Fiber: 2 g.

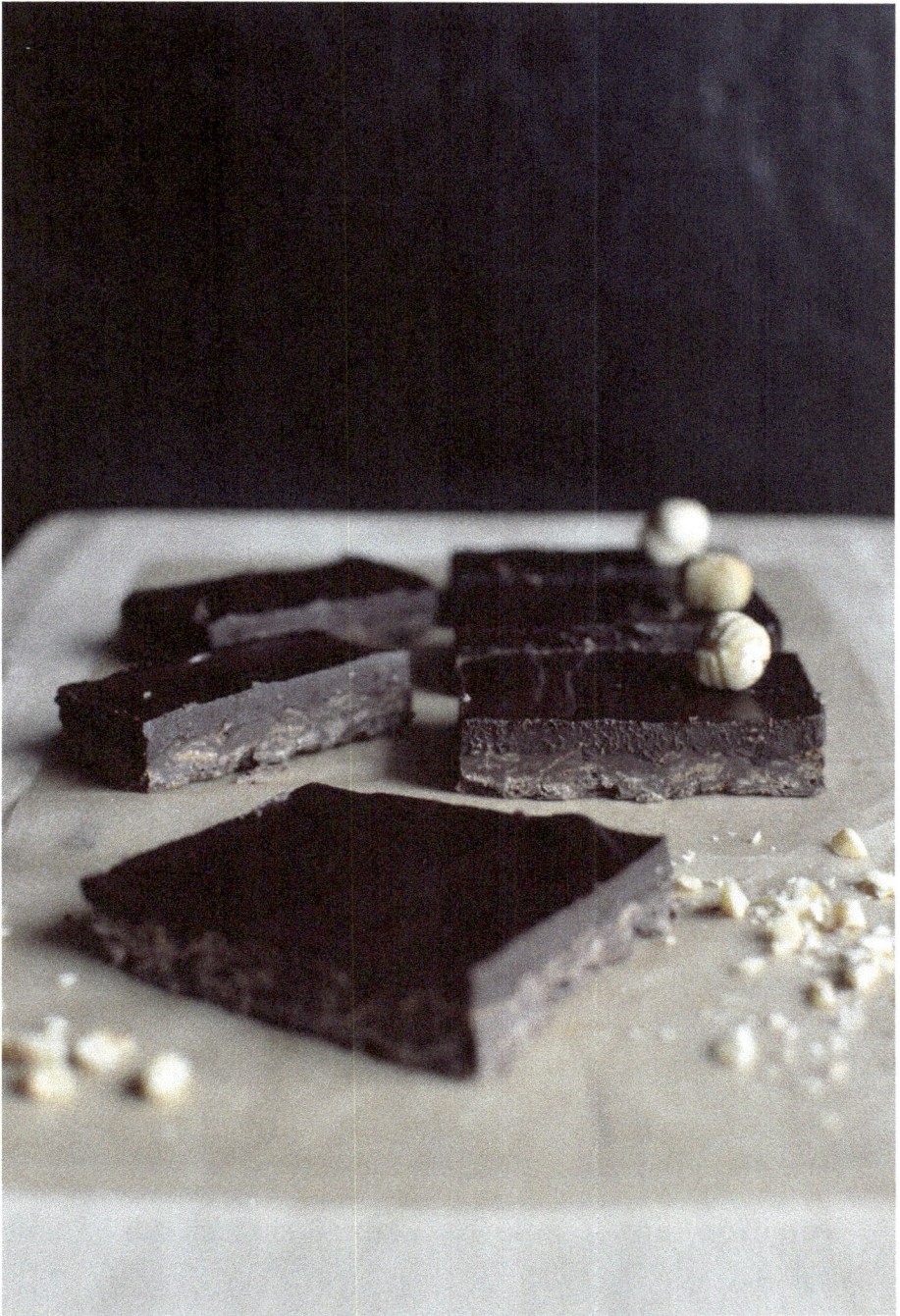

Chocolate Fudge

Servings: 16

Cooking Time: 15 Minutes

Ingredients:

- 8 oz. chocolate chips, unsweetened
- 1/2 cup peanut butter

Directions:

1. Cover an 8 square inch pan with baking lining and set to the side.
2. Heat a saucepan to melt the chocolate chips until liquefied. Then blend in the peanut butter until the batter is smooth.
3. Distribute to the prepped pan and level out with a rubber scraper
4. Put the fudge into the freezer for 10 minutes to firm.
5. Slice and enjoy!
6. Tricks and Tips:
7. If you have an allergy to peanuts, you can substitute coconut butter, almond butter or sun butter instead.
8. There are many varieties that you can experiment with by adding your favorite ingredients. Try shredded coconut, chopped walnuts or chia seeds.

Nutrition Info: 3 grams ;Net Carbs: 8.1 grams ;Fat: 8 grams ;Calories: 114

Lemon Bars

Servings: 8

Cooking Time: 60 Minutes

Ingredients:

- 1 3/4 cups almond flour
- 3 lemons
- 1 cup erythritol sweetener
- 1/2 cup unsalted butter, melted
- 3 eggs

Directions:

1. Set oven to 350 degrees F and let preheat.
2. Place 1 cup flour, sweetener, and butter in a bowl and stir until mixed.
3. Spoon the mixture evenly into 8 by 8-inch baking dish, lined with parchment paper, and press and spread evenly.
4. Place baking dish into the oven and bake for 20 minutes.
5. When done, place baking dish on wire rack and cool for 10 minutes.
6. Zest one lemon, add to bowl, then add the juice of all lemons and add remaining ingredients.
7. Stir until combined, then spoon the mixture into the baking dish and spread evenly.

8. Place the baking dish into the oven to bake for 25 minutes or until set and top is nicely browned.

9. Slice and serve with lemon slices.

Nutrition Info: Calories: 272 Cal, Carbs: 4 g, Fat: 26 g, Protein: 8 g, Fiber: 3 g.

Sesame Bars

Servings: 16

Cooking Time: 15 Minutes

Ingredients:

- 1 14 cups sesame seeds
- 10 drops liquid stevia
- 12 tsp vanilla
- 14 cup unsweetened applesauce
- 34 cup coconut butter
- Pinch of salt

Directions:

1. Preheat the oven to 350 F o C.
2. Spray a baking dish with cooking spray and set aside.
3. In a large bowl, add applesauce, coconut butter, vanilla, liquid stevia, and sea salt and stir until well combined.
4. Add sesame seeds and stir to coat.
5. Pour mixture into a prepared baking dish and bake in preheated oven for 10-1minutes.
6. Remove from oven and set aside to cool completely.
7. Place in refrigerator for 1 hour.
8. Cut into pieces and serve.

Nutrition Info: Per Servings: Net Carbs: 2.4g; Calories: 136 Total Fat: 12.4g; Saturated Fat: 6.8g Protein: 2.8g; Carbs: 5.7g; Fiber: 3.3g; Sugar: 1.2g; Fat 83% Protein Carbs 8%

Lemon

Servings: 8

Cooking Time: 1 Hour

Ingredients:

- 1 cup sweetener, confectioner
- 3 large eggs
- 1/4 tsp. salt
- 1 3/4 cups almond flour
- 3 medium lemons
- 1/2 cup butter, melted

Directions:

1. Set your stove to the temperature of 350° Fahrenheit. Cover an 8-inch cake pan with baking paper and set to the side.

2. In a big dish, blend 1 cup of the almond flour and butter until fully incorporated. Add the sweetener (1/4 cup) and salt (1/8 teaspoon) and combine completely.

3. Push the batter squarely into the prepped pan and heat for 20 minutes. Remove and set on a heat resistant surface while mixing the filling.

4. Zest 1 lemon in a dish and add the juice from all 3 lemons. Add the remaining 3/cup almond flour and mix well.Add 1 egg and cream into the mixture, repeating for all the eggs.

5. Finally, add the sweetener (3/4 cup) and salt (1/8 teaspoon) and incorporate thoroughly.
6. Transfer the filling to the cooled baking pan and heat in the stove for 25 more minutes.
7. Remove and dust the top with sweetener and garnish with a slice of lemon, if preferred.

Nutrition Info: grams ;Net Carbs: 4 grams ;Fat: 26 grams ;Calories: 272

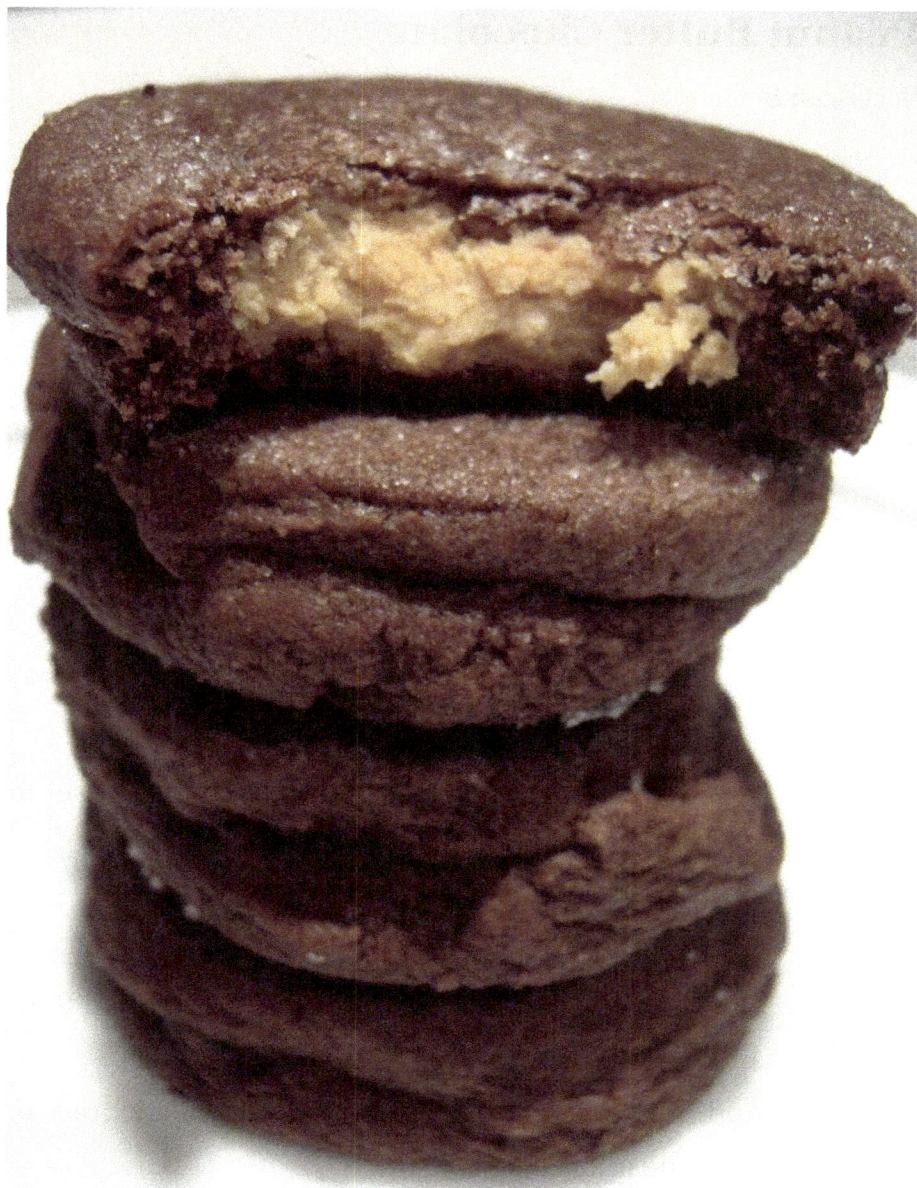

Peanut Butter Chocolate

Servings: 8

Cooking Time: 2 Hours 10 Minutes

Ingredients:

- For the bars:
- 1/2 cup peanut butter
- 3/4 cup almond flour
- 1/4 cup Swerve Icing Sugar Style
- 2 oz. butter
- 1/2 tsp. vanilla extract, sugar-free
- For the topping:
- 4 oz. chocolate chips, sugar-free

Directions:

1. Layer baking paper on a 6-inch baking pan and set to the side.
2. On low/medium heat, melt the chocolate chips in a saucepan.
3. Use a food processor on high to whip the almond flour and butter.
4. Add the peanut butter, Swerve and vanilla extract to combine fully.
5. Use a rubber scraper to smooth out in the prepped pan and empty the melted chocolate on top.
6. Cool in the refrigerator for 2 hours. Slice and enjoy!

7. Tricks and Tips:

8. If you leave in the refrigerator, the flavors will become richer and the sugar will not be so granulated.

Nutrition Info: 7 grams ;Net Carbs: 4 grams ;Fat: 8 grams ;Calories: 246

Coconut Peanut Butter Bars

Servings: 12

Cooking Time: 10 Minutes

Ingredients:

- 1 cup unsweetened shredded coconut
- ½ tsp vanilla
- 1 tbsp swerve
- 1 cup creamy peanut butter
- ¼ cup butter
- Pinch of salt

Directions:

1. Add butter in microwave safe bowl and microwave until butter is melted.
2. Add peanut butter and stir well.
3. Add sweetener, vanilla, and salt and stir.
4. Add shredded coconut and mix until well combined.
5. Transfer mixture into the greased baking dish and spread evenly.
6. Place in refrigerator for 1 hour.
7. Slice and serve.

Nutrition Info: Per Servings: Net Carbs: 3.; Calories: 221 Total Fat: 20g; Saturated Fat: 9.4g Protein: 6.1g; Carbs: 6.4g; Fiber: 2.6g; Sugar: 2.7g; Fat 82% Protein 12% Carbs 6

Chocolate Peppermint Bars

Servings: 16

Cooking Time:20 Minutes

Ingredients:

- Base:
- 1 cup ground almonds
- 1 cup finely chopped walnuts
- 4 oz butter, melted
- 3 Tbsp unsweetened cocoa powder
- 1 tsp baking powder
- ½ tsp Stevia/your preferred keto sweetener
- Filling:
- 2 cups unsweetened dried coconut (small pieces, not thread)
- 2 Tbsp butter, melted
- 2 Tbsp full fat cream
- 1 ½ tsp peppermint essence
- ½ tsp Stevia/your preferred keto sweetener
- Topping:
- 8 oz 72% cocoa dark chocolate
- ½ cup heavy cream
- Pinch of salt

Directions:

1. Preheat the oven to 360 degrees Fahrenheit and line a brownie pan with baking paper
2. Combine all of the base ingredients until fully combined and press the mixture into your prepared brownie pan
3. Pop the pan into the oven and bake the base for about 20 minutes, leave to cool completely
4. Stir together the filling ingredients until combined, and spread the mixture over your baked and cooled base and pop into the fridge as you make the topping
5. Make the topping: place the chocolate, cream and salt into a heatproof bowl over a saucepan of simmering water and stir as the chocolate melts into the cream, leave to cool slightly
6. Pour the melted chocolate mixture over the cooled filling and spread it out with a spatula
7. Place the pan into the fridge to chill before cutting into 16 bars

Nutrition Info: Calories: 296;Fat: 2grams ;Protein: 4 grams ;Total carbs: 8 grams ;Net carbs: 3 grams

Almond Butter Bars

Servings: 6

Cooking Time: 27 Minutes

Ingredients:

- 1 cup raw almonds, chopped
- 1 cup slivered almonds
- 1 cup sugar free coconut flakes, tightly packed
- 1 large egg
- 4 tbsp monk fruit
- 2 tbsp almond butter
- 1 tbsp coconut oil
- 3/4 tsp sea salt
- 1/4 cup stevia sweetened chocolate chips

Directions:

1. Let your oven preheat at 375 degrees F. Layer an 8-inch pan with wax paper.
2. Spread chopped almond, coconut flakes and slivered almonds on separate baking sheets.
3. Toast the chopped almonds for 12 minutes, slivered almonds for 5 minutes and coconut shreds for 4 minutes.
4. Whisk egg with monk fruit in a suitable bowl.
5. Melt almond butter with coconut oil in a small bowl by heating in a microwave for 30 seconds.

6. Add this butter into the egg mixture then mix well.

7. Toss in all the nuts, salt, and coconut. Then stir in chocolate chips.

8. Add this mixture to the pan and press it firmly.

9. Bake the batter for 15 minutes at 350 degrees F.

10. Allow it to cool the slice.

11. Serve.

Nutrition Info: Per Servings: Calories 220 Total Fat 20.1 g Saturated Fat 7.4 g Cholesterol 132 mg Total Carbs 63 g Sugar 0.4 g Fiber 2.4 g Sodium 157 mg Potassium 42 mg Protein 6.1 g

Flavors Pumpkin Bars

Servings: 18

Cooking Time: 10 Minutes

Ingredients:

- 1 tbsp coconut flour
- ½ tsp cinnamon
- 2 tsp pumpkin pie spice
- 1 tsp liquid stevia
- ½ cup erythritol
- 15 oz can pumpkin puree
- 15 oz can unsweetened coconut milk
- 16 oz cocoa butter

Directions:

1. Line baking dish with parchment paper and set aside.
2. Melt cocoa butter in a small saucepan over low heat.
3. Add pumpkin puree and coconut milk and stir well.
4. Add remaining ingredients and whisk well.
5. Stir the mixture continuously until mixture thickens.
6. Once the mixture thickens then pour it into prepared baking dish and place in the refrigerator for 2 hours.
7. Slice and serve.

Nutrition Info: Per Servings: Net Carbs: 5.; Calories: 282; Total Fat: 28.1g; Saturated Fat: 17.1gProtein: 1.3g; Carbs: 9.5g; Fiber: 3.7g; Sugar: 4g; Fat 89% Protein 2% Carbs 9%

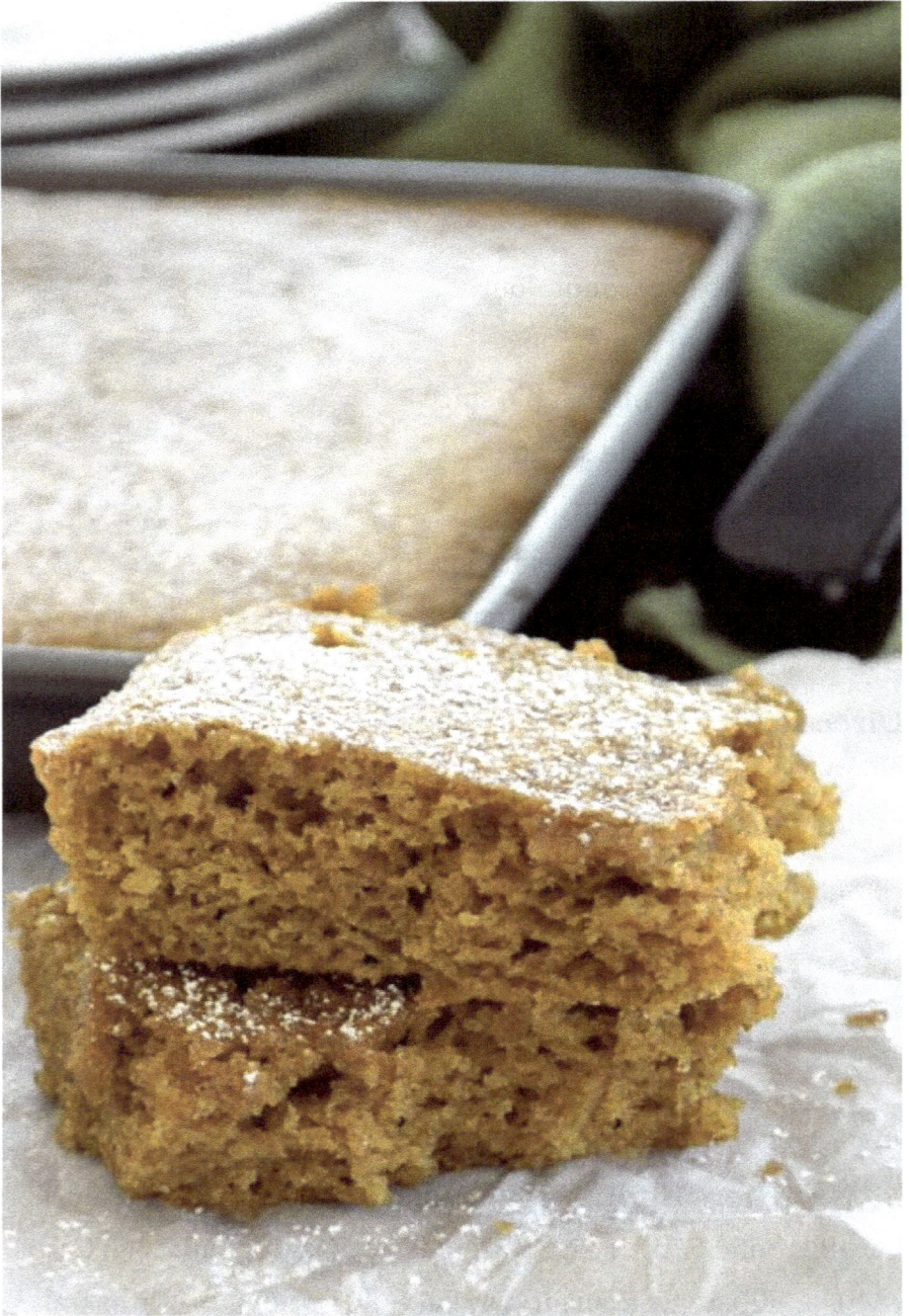

Peanut Butter Chocolate Bars

Servings: 8

Cooking Time: 1 Hour And 5 Minutes

Ingredients:

- For the Bars:
- 3/4 cup almond flour
- 1/4 cup Swerve Sweetener
- 1/2 teaspoon Vanilla extract, unsweetened
- 2-ounce unsalted butter
- 1/2 cup peanut butter
- For the Topping:
- 1/2 cup chocolate chips, sugar-free

Directions:

1. Place all the ingredients for bars in a large bowl, mix well and then spread evenly into a 6-inch pan.
2. Place chocolate chips in a heatproof bowl and microwave for 45 seconds or until melt.
3. Stir well, then spread chocolate on top of bars and refrigerate for 1 hour or more until thickened.
4. Cut into even pieces and serve.

Nutrition Info: Calories: 246 Cal, Carbs: 7 g, Fat: 23 g, Protein: 7 g, Fiber: 3 g.

Protein Bars

Servings: 8

Cooking Time: 10 Minutes

Ingredients:

- 2 scoops vanilla protein powder
- ½ tsp cinnamon
- 15 drops liquid stevia
- ¼ cup coconut oil, melted
- 1 cup almond butter
- Pinch of salt

Directions:

1. In a bowl, mix together all ingredients until well combined.
2. Transfer bar mixture into a baking dish and press down evenly.
3. Place in refrigerator until firm.
4. Slice and serve.

Nutrition Info: Per Servings: Net Carbs: 0.2g; Calories: 99 Total Fat: 8g; Saturated Fat: 6g Protein: 7.2g; Carbs: 0.6g; Fiber: 0.4g; Sugar: 0.2g; Fat 71% Protein 28% Carbs 1%

No-bake Keto Chocolate Peppermint Cookie Bars

Servings: 20

Cooking Time: 10 Minutes

Ingredients:

- 6 cups shredded coconut
- 4 tablespoons ghee
- 8-12 drops food grade peppermint essential oil
- 6 teaspoons vanilla extract
- 4 tablespoons MitoSweet or granulated erythritol / monk fruit blend
- ¾ cup collagen protein
- 4 teaspoons organic chlorella powder
- ¼ teaspoon salt
- For chocolate drizzle:
- 4 tablespoons cacao powder
- 2 teaspoons vanilla extract
- 6 tablespoons ghee or coconut oil, melted
- 2 tablespoons MitoSweet or granulated erythritol / monk fruit blend or 30 drops liquid stevia

Directions:

1. To make cookie bars: Add coconut into a blender and blend on medium or high speed until finely chopped.

2. Add ghee, peppermint oil, vanilla, sweetener, chlorella and salt and blend until well incorporated.

3. Add collagen and set the blender to low speed. Pulse for a few seconds until well incorporated.

4. Line 2 loaf pans with parchment paper.

5. Divide the mixture equally among the pans. Press well into the pans.

6. Place in the freezer for about 45 minutes to an hour until set.

7. Meanwhile, make the chocolate drizzle as follows: Add cacao, vanilla, sweetener and coconut oil into a bowl and whisk until well combined.

8. Make 10 equal slices from each loaf pan. Trickle chocolate mixture over the bars.

9. Place in the freezer until chocolate sets.

10. Refrigerate until used. Remove from the molds and serve.

11. Leftovers can be stored in an airtight container in the refrigerator. These can keep for 4 – 5 days.

Nutrition Info: Per Servings: Calories: 197.6 kcal, Fat: 15.7 g, Carbohydrates: 4.1 g, Protein: 11.9 g

Chocolate Chips Granola Bars

Servings: 16

Cooking Time: 30 Minutes

Ingredients:

- 1/3 cup goji berries
- 1/4 cup flax meal
- 1/4 cup chocolate chips, stevia sweetened
- 1/2 teaspoon ground ginger
- 3 tablespoons swerve sweetener
- 1/3 cup sukrin syrup
- 1 teaspoon cinnamon
- 1/3 cup pumpkin seeds
- 1/3 cup sunflower seeds
- 2 cups sliced almonds
- 1/2 cup walnuts
- 1/2 cup pecans
- 2 tablespoons melted butter, unsalted

Directions:

1. Set oven to 350 degrees F and let preheat.
2. In the meantime, line a 13 by 9-inch baking dish with parchment paper and then grease with oil, set aside until required.
3. Place almonds in a food processor and pulse until chopped.

4. Tip almonds in a bowl, add remaining ingredients except for butter and syrup and stir well.

5. Then add butter and stir until mixed.

6. Add syrup and stir well and spoon the mixture into prepared baking dish.

7. Spread the mixture evenly, then cover with a wax paper and press granola with a flat-bottomed glass.

8. Place the baking dish into the oven and bake for 15 to 20 minutes or until edges begin to brown.

9. When done, cool the dish at room temperature for 10 minutes and then lift the parchment paper to take out granola.

10. Let granola cool completely, then cut into 16 bars and serve.

Nutrition Info: Calories: 307 Cal, Carbs: 10 g, Fat: 27 g, Protein: 6 g, Fiber: 6 g.

Peanut Butter Bars

Servings: 9

Cooking Time: 30 Minutes

Ingredients:

- 2 eggs
- 1 tbsp coconut flour
- ¼ cup almond flour
- ½ cup erythritol
- ½ cup butter softened
- ½ cup peanut butter

Directions:

1. Spray 9*9-inch baking pan with cooking spray and set aside.
2. In a bowl, beat together butter, eggs, and peanut butter until well combined.
3. Add dry ingredients and mix until a smooth batter is formed.
4. Spread batter evenly in prepared baking pan.
5. Bake at 3 F 180 C for 30 minutes.
6. Slice and serve.

Nutrition Info: Per Servings: Net Carbs: 2.8g; Calories: 213; Total Fat: 20.2g; Saturated Fat: 8.6g Protein: 5.8g; Carbs: 4.5g; Fiber: 1.; Sugar: 1.7g; Fat 85% Protein 10% Carbs 5%

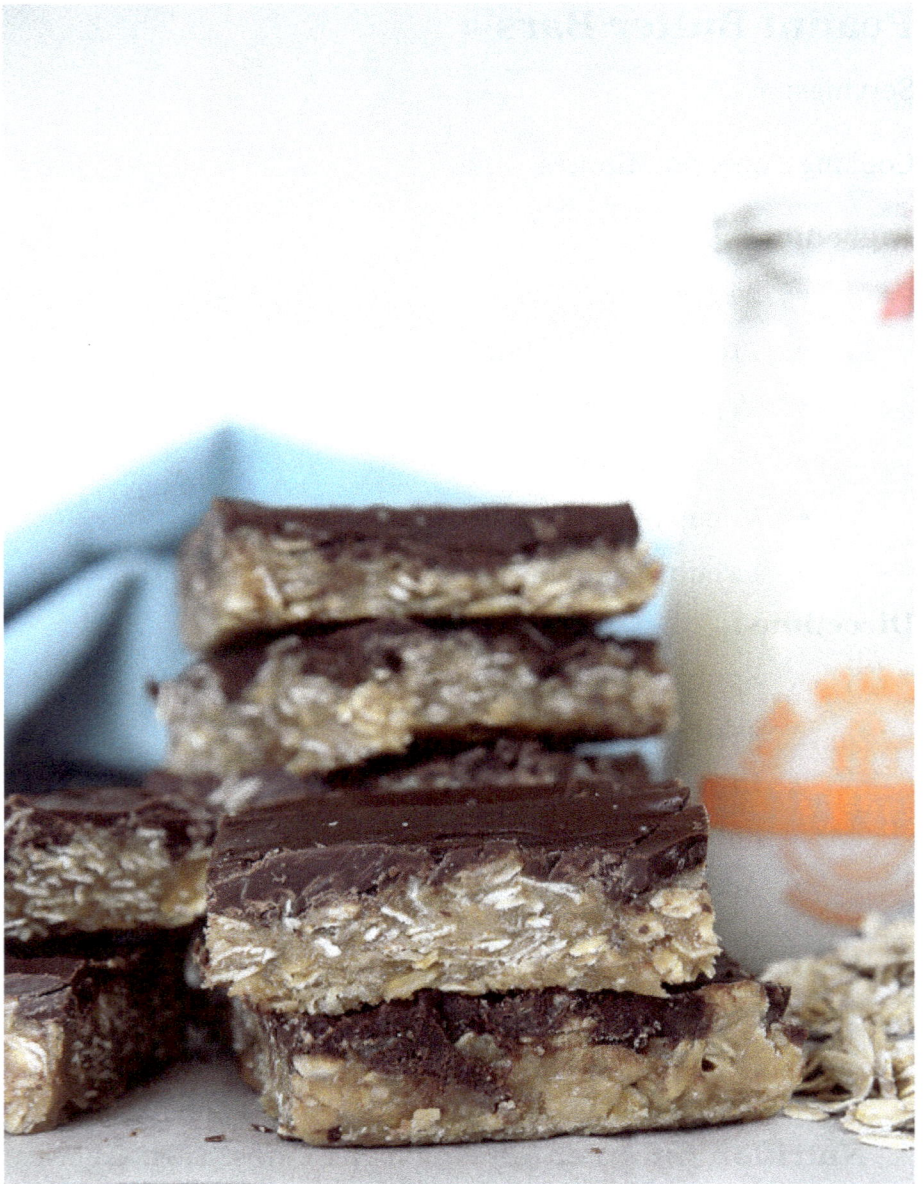

36

Keto Protein Bar

Servings: 6

Cooking Time: 0 Minute

Ingredients:

- 1 cup of nut butter
- 4 tbsps. of coconut oil (melted)
- 2 scoops of vanilla protein
- 10-15 drops of vanilla stevia
- ½ tsp of pink salt
- Optional
- 4 tbsps. of sugar-free chocolate chips
- 1 tsp of cinnamon

Directions:

1. Toss all the ingredients together in a suitable bowl.
2. Spread this mixture into a loaf pan.
3. Place the pan in the freezer then cut it into small bars.
4. Serve.

Nutrition Info: Per Servings: Calories 179 Total Fat 17 g Saturated Fat 8 g Cholesterol 0 mg Total Carbs 4.8 g Sugar 3.6 g Fiber 0.8 g Sodium 43 mg Potassium 15 mg Protein 5.6 g

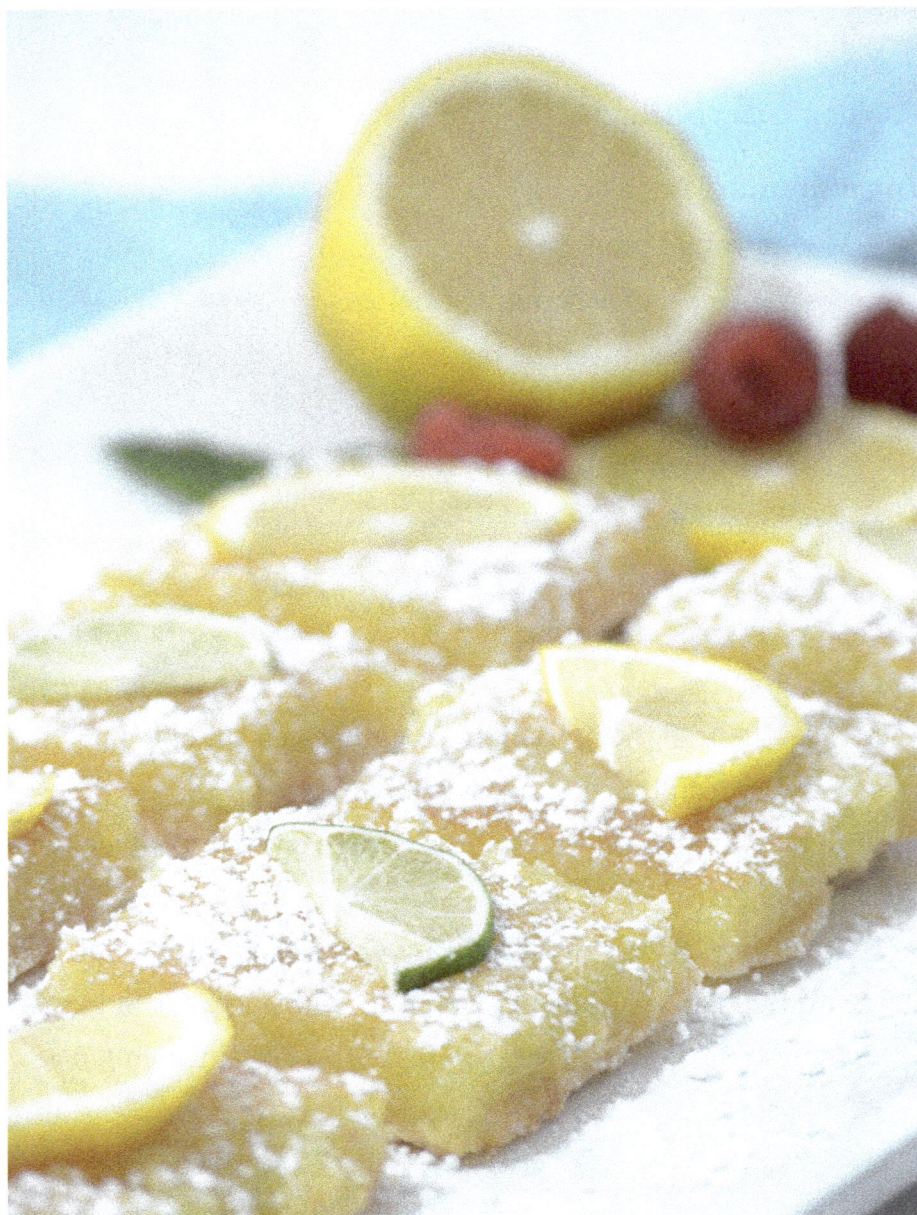

Easy Lemon Bars

Servings: 8

Cooking Time: 40 Minutes

Ingredients:

- 4 eggs
- 13 cup erythritol
- 2 tsp baking powder
- 2 cups almond flour
- 1 lemon zest
- ¼ cup fresh lemon juice
- ½ cup butter softened
- ½ cup sour cream

Directions:

1. Preheat the oven to 350 F 0 C.
2. Line 9*6-inch baking pan with parchment paper. Set aside.
3. In a bowl, beat eggs until frothy.
4. Add butter and sour cream and beat until well combined.
5. Add sweetener, lemon zest, and lemon juice and blend well.
6. Add baking powder and almond flour and mix until well combined.

7. Transfer batter in a prepared baking pan and spread evenly.

8. Bake in preheated oven for 35-40 minutes.

9. Remove from oven and allow to cool completely.

10. Slice and serve.

Nutrition Info: Per Servings: Net Carbs: 4.9g; Calories: 329; Total Fat: 30.8g; Saturated Fat: 10.9g Protein: 9.5g; Carbs: 8.2g; Fiber: 3.3g; Sugar: 1.5g; Fat 84% Protein Carbs 5%

Keto Almond Milk Bars

Servings: 8

Cooking Time: 32 Minutes

Ingredients:

- Crust
- 1 large egg
- 1 cup almond flour
- 1/4 teaspoon salt
- 2 tablespoons butter, unsalted
- Condensed Milk
- Pinch of salt
- 1/2 cup heavy cream
- 1/2 cup Swerve
- 1/2 cup butter, unsalted
- 1 teaspoon vanilla essence
- Top Layer
- 1 cup sugar free shredded coconut
- 9 oz sugar free Chocolate Chips
- 1 cup pecan, chopped

Directions:

1. For the crust
2. Let your oven preheat at 300 degrees F.
3. Add and mix all the crust ingredients in a bowl until it forms a dough ball.

41

4. Spread this dough in an 8-inch baking pan and poke holes in it using a fork.

5. Bake the dough crust for 20 minutes until golden.

6. For the condensed milk:

7. Mix and heat all the condensed milk ingredients in a cooking pot.

8. Let it boil for 5 minutes with constant stirring.

9. Turn off the heat once this mixture thickens.

10. To assemble:

11. Toss pecan, chopped with chocolate chips and coconut.

12. Spread this mixture over the baked crust then pour the condensed milk over it.

13. Bake again for 7 minutes.

14. Refrigerate it for 1 hour.

15. Slice into small bars.

16. Serve.

Nutrition Info: Per Servings: Calories 358 Total Fat 35.2 g Saturated Fat 15.2 g Cholesterol 69 mg Total Carbs 7.4 g Sugar 1.1 g Fiber 3.5 g Sodium mg Potassium 114 mg Protein 5.5 g

Lemon Egg Bars

Servings: 8

Cooking Time: 45 Minutes

Ingredients:

- 1/2 cup butter, melted
- 1 3/4 cups almond flour
- 1 cup erythritol, powdered
- Juice from 3 medium lemons
- 3 large eggs

Directions:

1. Take an 8-inch baking pan and line it with parchment paper.
2. Whisk butter with almond flour, erythritol, and salt in a suitable bowl.
3. Transfer the crumbly batter to a pan and press it firmly.
4. Bake the crust for 20 mins in the preheated oven at 350 degrees F.
5. Once the crust is done, allow it to cool for 10 minutes at room temperature.
6. Mix rest of the ingredients in a separate bowl.
7. Pour it over the baked crust and spread it evenly.
8. Again bake it for 25 minutes in the oven at the same temperature.

9. Remove the pan and slice the bars.

10. Garnish with erythritol.

11. Serve and enjoy.

Nutrition Info: Calories 282 ;Total Fat 25.1 g ;Saturated Fat 8.8 g ;Cholesterol 100 mg ;Sodium 117 mg ;Total Carbs 9.4 g ;Sugar 0.7 g ;Fiber 3.2 g ;Protein 8 g

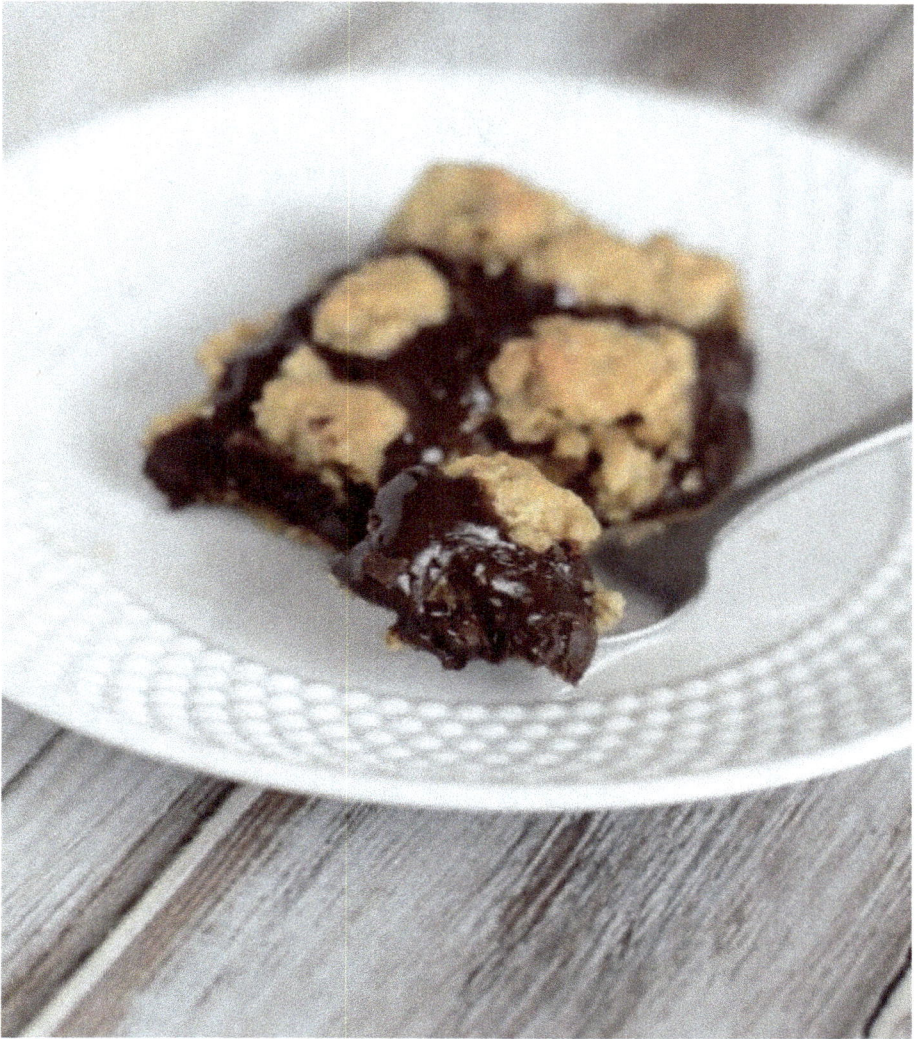

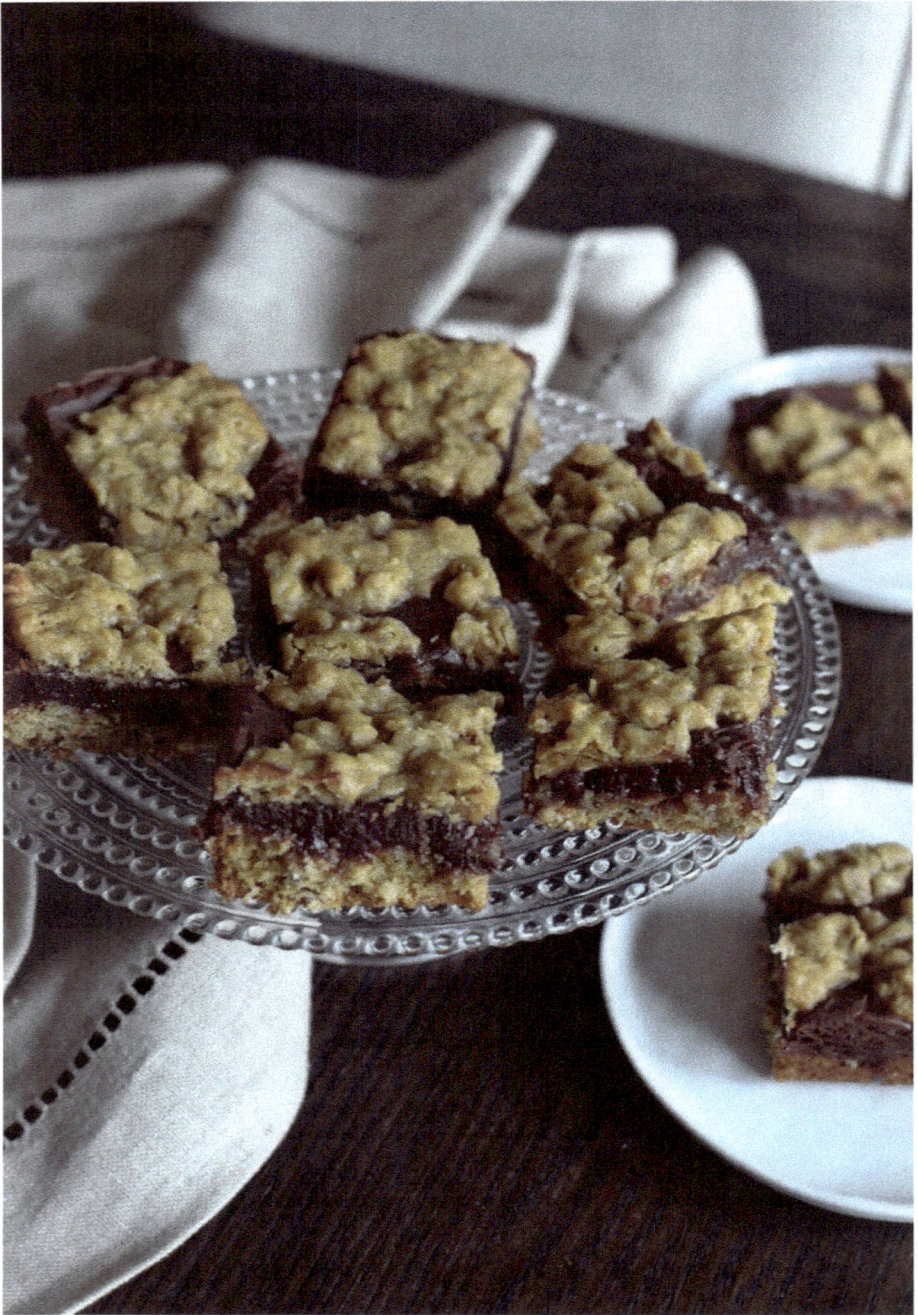

Butter Fudge Bars

Servings: 36

Cooking Time: 10 Minutes

Ingredients:

- 1 cup unsweetened peanut butter
- 12 cup whey protein powder
- 1 tsp stevia
- 1 cup erythritol
- 8 oz cream cheese
- 1 tsp vanilla
- 1 cup butter

Directions:

1. Spray baking pan with cooking spray and line with parchment paper. Set aside.
2. Melt butter and cream cheese in a saucepan over medium heat.
3. Add peanut butter and stir to combine.
4. Remove pan from heat.
5. Add remaining ingredients and blend until well combined.
6. Pour mixture into the prepared pan and spread evenly.
7. Place in refrigerator for 1-2 hours or until set.
8. Slice and serve.

Nutrition Info: Per Servings: Net Carbs: 1.2g; Calories: 111; Total Fat: 11g; Saturated Fat: 5.3g Protein: 2.3g; Carbs: 1.6g; Fiber: 0.4g; Sugar: 0.5g; Fat 88% Protein 8% Carbs 4%

Keto Coconut Bars

Servings: 6

Cooking Time: 0 Minute

Ingredients:

- 3 cups desiccated coconut sugar free
- 1/3 cup coconut cream
- 1/2 cup sugar-free syrup
- 4 tbsp coconut oil
- 1 oz sugar-free chocolate minimum

Directions:

1. Add everything to a blender and blend them together on high speed.
2. Layer an 8x5 inch baking pan with wax paper.
3. Spread the coconut mixture into the prepared pan.
4. Press the mixture with your hand to smoothen out the surface.
5. Refrigerate this mixture for 1minutes.
6. Slice it into square pieces.
7. Add chocolate to a bowl and melt it in the microwave.
8. Drizzle the melted chocolate over the coconut bars.
9. Return the bars to your refrigerator for 10 minutes.
10. Serve.

Nutrition Info: Per Servings: Calories 214 Total Fat 19 g Saturated Fat 5.8 g Cholesterol 15 mg Total Carbs 6.5 g Sugar 1.9 g Fiber 2.1 g Sodium 123 mg Potassium mg Protein 6.5 g

Keto Chocolate Bar

Servings: 6

Cooking Time: 0 Minute

Ingredients:

- 3 oz Cocoa butter
- 2 1/2 oz Sugar free baking chocolate
- 6 tbsp erythritol powder
- 2 tbsp Inulin
- 1/4 tsp Sunflower lecithin
- 1/8 tsp Sea salt
- 1 tsp Vanilla essence

Directions:

1. Melt chocolate with cocoa butter in a double boiler on low heat.
2. Mix chocolate mixture with erythritol in a saucepan.
3. Stir in inulin, salt and sunflower lecithin.
4. Heat this mixture until smooth then turn off the heat.
5. Stir in vanilla essence and mix well.
6. Divide this mixture into a bar mold tray.
7. Place the bar tray in the refrigerator for 30 minutes.
8. Serve.

Nutrition Info: Per Servings: Calories 331 Total Fat 32.g Saturated Fat 6.1 g Cholesterol 10 mg Total Carbs 9.1 g Sugar

2.8 g Fiber 0.8 g Sodium 18 mg Potassium 37 mg Protein 4.4 g

Samoa Cookie Bars

Servings: 6

Cooking Time: 30 Minutes

Ingredients:

- Crust
- 1/4 cup swerve
- 1 1/4 cups almond flour
- 1/4 tsp salt
- 1/4 cup butter, melted
- filling and drizzle
- 2 tbsp butter, melted
- 4 ounces sugar-free chocolate, diced
- caramel filling
- 3 tbsp butter
- 1/4 cup swerve brown
- 3/4 cup heavy whipping cream
- 1 1/2 cups shredded coconut
- 1/4 cup mocha sweet
- 1/2 tsp vanilla essence
- 1/4 tsp salt

Directions:

1. Crust
2. Let your oven preheat at 3 degrees F.

3. Mix almond flour with salt and sweetener in a medium bowl.
4. Stir in melted butter then spread this mixture in an 8-inch baking pan.
5. Press the mixture into the pan and bake it for 18 minutes.
6. Chocolate Filling/Drizzle
7. Melt chocolate with coconut oil in a glass bowl by heating in a microwave for 30 seconds.
8. Spread half of that melted chocolate over the baked crust.
9. Coconut Filling
10. Add coconut to a skillet and toast it until golden brown.
11. Melt butter in a saucepan with sweeteners.
12. Cook this mixture for 5 minutes until golden.
13. Remove it from the heat then stir in salt, cream, and vanilla.
14. Cook this mixture until it bubbles.
15. Gently stir in toasted coconut.
16. Add this mixture into the crust and allow it to cool for 1 hour.
17. Cut it into small squares.
18. Drizzle the remaining chocolate over them.
19. Serve.

Nutrition Info: Per Servings: Calories 313 Total Fat 28.4 g Saturated Fat 12.1 g Cholesterol 27 mg Total Carbs 9.2 g Sugar 3.1 g Fiber 4.6 g Sodium 39 mg Potassium 185 mg Protein 8.1 g

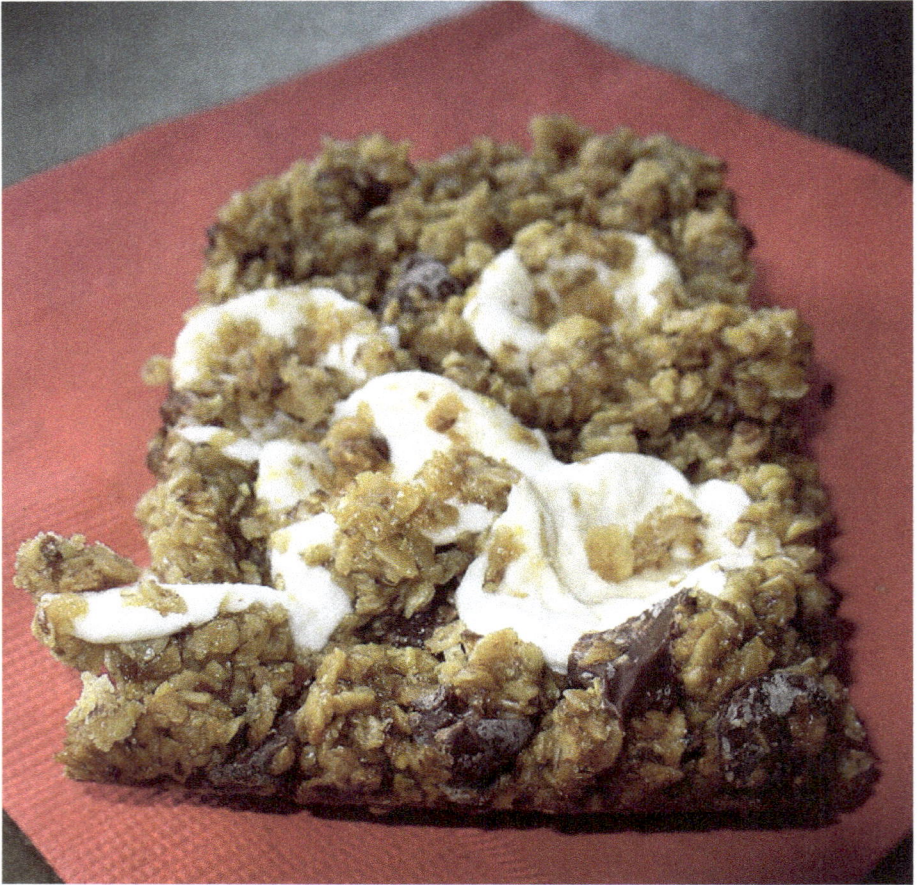

Chocolate Dipped Granola Bars

Servings: 4

Cooking Time: 20 Minutes

Ingredients:

- 1 egg
- 3 tablespoons coconut oil
- 1 ½ oz. almonds
- 1 oz. sesame seeds
- 1¼ teaspoon flaxseed
- 1 oz. coconut, shredded, unsweetened
- 1 ½ oz. walnuts
- 1 oz. sugar-free dark chocolate
- 1 oz. pumpkin seeds
- 2 tablespoons tahini
- 1 teaspoon cinnamon, ground
- ½ pinch sea salt
- ½ teaspoon vanilla essence
- 1 ½ oz. sugar-free dark chocolate

Directions:

1. Let your oven preheat at 350 degrees F.
2. Coarsely grind all the ingredients except chocolate in a food processor.
3. Spread the ground mixture in a suitable baking pan layered with wax paper.

4. Transfer the baking pan to the middle rack of the oven to bake for 20 minutes.
5. Once ready, remove the base of the bar from the pan and allow it to cool at room temperature.
6. Slice it into small squares and place them over a wire rack.
7. Melt the chocolate in a bowl in a microwave.
8. Pour this melt over the bars evenly.
9. Place the bars over a baking sheet.
10. Refrigerate them for 20 minutes until the chocolate has set.
11. Serve and enjoy.

Nutrition Info: Calories 313 ;Total Fat 28.4 g ;Saturated Fat 1 g ;Cholesterol 27 mg ;Sodium 39 mg ;Total Carbs 9.2 g ;Sugar 3.1 g ;Fiber 4.6 g ;Protein 8.1 g

Flourless Keto Chocolate Cake

Servings: 8

Cooking Time: 30 Minutes

Ingredients:

- ¾ cup butter
- 1 teaspoon vanilla extract
- 3 large eggs
- 12 ounce sugar-free baker's chocolate (you can use stevia sweetened chocolate)
- 1/8 teaspoon salt
- ¼ cup erythritol + extra to sprinkle

Directions:

1. Grease a 6-inch springform pan with cooking spray. Place a round sheet of parchment paper in it.
2. Melt chocolate and butter in double boiler. Add 1-cup erythritol and mix until dissolved. Remove from the double boiler.
3. Add vanilla and salt and beat with an electric hand mixer on low speed until well combined. Add eggs, one at a time and beat well each time. Add erythritol and beat well. All this is done on low speed.
4. Place the springform pan over a baking sheet.
5. Bake in a preheated oven at 3° F for about 20-25 minutes and not longer than this. The cake will look

undercooked. The internal temperature of the cake should show 140° with a cooking thermometer. When this temperature is reached, remove the cake from the oven. Cool completely in the pan.

6. Place the pan in the refrigerator for 8-9 hours.

7. Remove from the refrigerator and place on your countertop for an hour. Remove from the pan and place on a serving platter.

8. Sprinkle some erythritol on top. Cut into slices and serve.

9. Leftovers can be stored in an airtight container in the refrigerator. These can keep for a week.

Nutrition Info: Per Servings: Calories: 179.5 kcal, Fat: 19 g, Carbohydrates: 0.1 g, Protein: 1.3 g

Fudgy Chocolate Cake

Servings: 12

Cooking Time: 30 Minutes

Ingredients:

- 6 eggs
- 1 ½ cup erythritol
- ½ cup almond flour
- 10.5 oz butter, melted
- 10.5 oz unsweetened chocolate, melted
- Pinch of salt

Directions:

1. Preheat the oven to 350 F 0 C.
2. Grease 8-inch spring-form cake pan with butter and set aside.
3. In a large bowl, beat eggs until foamy.
4. Add sweetener and stir well.
5. Add melted butter, chocolate, almond flour, and salt and stir until combined.
6. Pour batter in the prepared cake pan and bake in preheated oven for 30 minutes.
7. Remove cake from oven and allow to cool completely.
8. Slice and serve.

Nutrition Info: Per Servings: Net Carbs: 4g; Calories: 360; Total Fat: 37.6g; Saturated Fat: 21.6g Protein: 7.2g;

Carbs: 8.6g; Fiber: 4.6g; Sugar: 0.6g; Fat % Protein 7% Carbs 3%

Keto Nutella Cake Roll

Servings: 6

Cooking Time: 10 Minutes

Ingredients:

- For cake:
- 3 large eggs
- 6 tablespoons powdered erythritol or Swerve
- ¼ teaspoon vanilla bean powder or 1 teaspoon vanilla extract
- A pinch sea salt or Himalayan pink salt
- ¾ cup almond flour
- For filling:
- ½ cup mascarpone cheese or creamed coconut milk, at room temperature
- ½ cup keto nutella
- For ganache coating:
- 3 tablespoons heavy whipping cream or coconut milk
- 1.75 ounces dark chocolate, broken into small pieces
- Stevia drops to taste (optional)
- 1 ½ tablespoons butter or virgin coconut oil
- ¼ teaspoon vanilla bean powder or 1 teaspoon vanilla extract

Directions:

1. Add eggs into a bowl. Whisk with an electric hand mixer until foamy.

2. Add salt and sweetener and continue beating.

3. Add flour and vanilla and fold gently.

4. Line a small baking sheet (half sheet pan) with heavy-duty parchment paper.

5. Spread the dough on the baking sheet.

6. Bake in a preheated oven at 350° F for about 8 to 10 minutes until light golden brown on top. Do not bake for long, or you will not be able to roll it, as it will break.

7. Place a sheet of parchment paper on your countertop. Invert the sponge cake onto the parchment paper. Take a slightly moist kitchen towel and cover the sponge cake with it for 2 to 3 minutes.

8. Carefully remove the parchment paper from the sponge cake.

9. Roll the warm sponge cake with the parchment paper, tightly. Set aside for a few minutes.

10. Meanwhile, make the filling by adding mascarpone cheese and nutella into a bowl. Whisk well.

11. Unroll the sponge on your countertop. Spread the nutella mixture evenly over the sponge, leaving about a ½ inch on the border.

12. Roll the sponge, without the parchment paper. Wrap the entire roll in parchment and chill for a few minutes.

13. In the meantime, make the ganache as follows: Place chocolate in a small bowl.

14. Add cream and butter into a saucepan. Place the saucepan over medium-high heat. When the mixture melts and well combined, turn off the heat and pour into the bowl of chocolate. Stir until the chocolate melts. Let it cool completely.

15. Remove the parchment paper. Spoon the ganache all over the top and sides of the nutella roll.

16. Chill until the ganache sets.

17. Slice and serve.

18. Leftovers can be stored in an airtight container in the refrigerator. The cake can keep for 5 days.

Nutrition Info: Per Servings: Calories: 314.2 kcal, Fat: 27.8 g, Carbohydrates: 7.5 g, Protein: 8.5 g

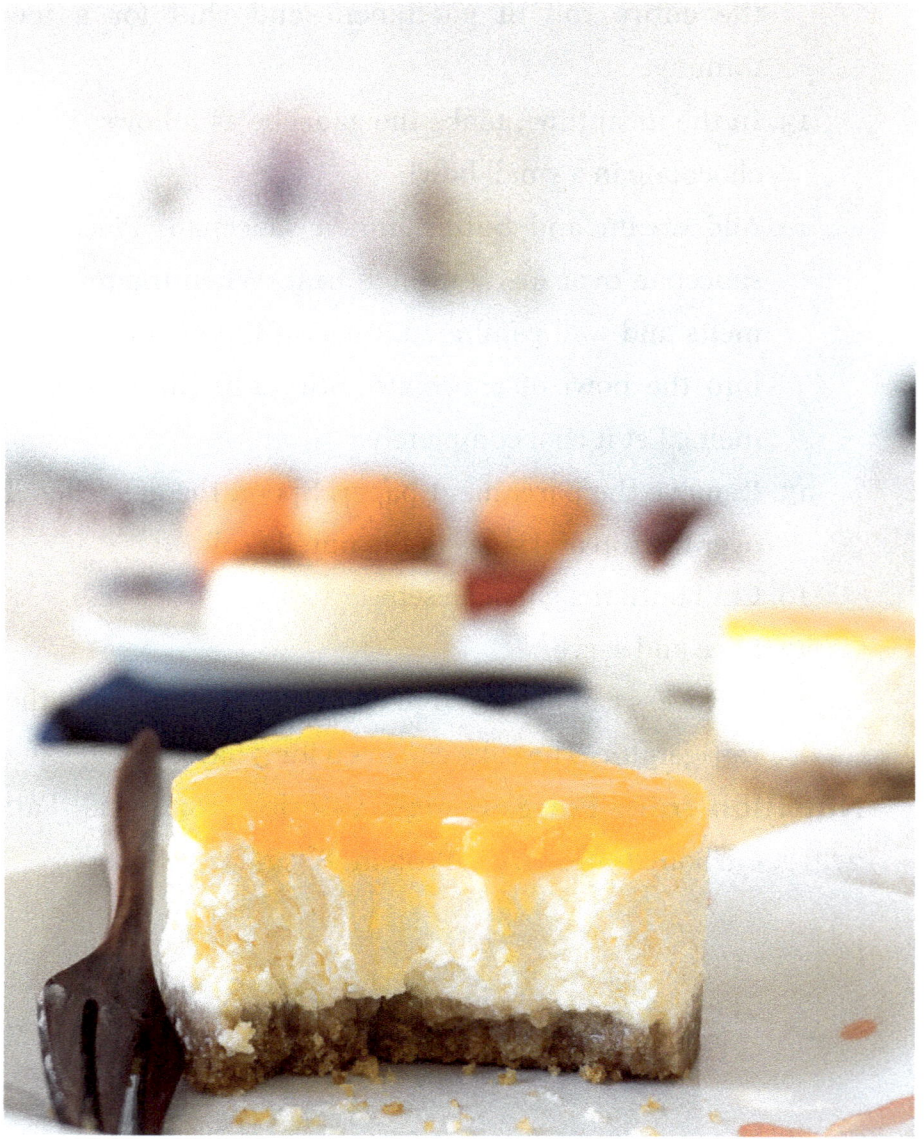

Lemon Cheesecake

Servings: 8

Cooking Time: 55 Minutes

Ingredients:

- 4 eggs
- 18 oz ricotta cheese
- 1 fresh lemon zest
- 2 tbsp swerve
- 1 fresh lemon juice

Directions:

1. Preheat the oven to 350 F 0 C.
2. Spray cake pan with cooking spray and set aside.
3. In a large bowl, beat ricotta cheese until smooth.
4. Add egg one by one and whisk well.
5. Add lemon juice, lemon zest, and swerve and mix well.
6. Transfer mixture into the prepared cake pan and bake for 50-55 minutes.
7. Remove cake from oven and set aside to cool completely.
8. Place cake in the fridge for 1-2 hours.
9. Slice and serve.

Nutrition Info: Per Servings: Net Carbs: 4.6g; Calories: 124; Total Fat: 7.3g; Saturated Fat: 3.9g Protein: 2g; Carbs:

4.8g; Fiber: 0.2g; Sugar: 0.7g; Fat 53% Protein 33% Carbs
14%

Keto Tres Leches Cake

Servings: 24

Cooking Time: 30 Minutes

Ingredients:

- For cake (dry ingredients):
- 1 cup coconut flour
- 1 cup Swerve granular sweetener, divided
- 1 teaspoon baking powder
- ¼ teaspoon salt
- For cake (wet ingredients):
- 12 eggs, separated
- 2 teaspoons vanilla extract
- 1 cup unsweetened coconut milk or almond milk
- 1 cup heavy cream
- 1 cup butter, melted, cooled
- 2 teaspoons vanilla stevia
- 1 cup half and half
- ½ cup brandy (optional)
- 1 cup Swerve sweetener
- For cannoli frosting:
- 16 ounces mascarpone cheese or cream cheese
- 16 ounces ricotta cheese
- Vanilla stevia drops to taste
- 8 ounces heavy whipping cream

Directions:

1. Line 2 springform pans (9 inches each) with parchment paper
2. Add all the dry ingredients into a bowl and stir.
3. Add whites into the mixing bowl of the stand mixer. Add Swerve and beat with the mixer until stiff peaks are formed. Set aside.
4. Add yolks and rest of the wet ingredients into another bowl and whisk well.
5. Add dry ingredients into the bowl of yolk mixture and fold gently.
6. Add whites and fold gently.
7. Divide the batter into the prepared pans.
8. Bake in a preheated oven at 350° F for about 30 minutes. Remove the pans from the oven and let the cake cool in the pans for 20 minutes.
9. Poke the cake at several places using a wooden skewer.
10. Add cream, coconut milk, brandy if using and half and half into a bowl and whisk well.
11. Drizzle this mixture into the holes. Let cake rest for 30 minutes.
12. Chill for a couple of hours.
13. Meanwhile, make the frosting as follows: Add all the ingredients for the frosting into the mixing bowl of the stand mixer. Whisk until creamy and thick.

14. Remove the cake from the pan by removing the sides of the pan.

15. Spread as much frosting as required over the cake. Store the remaining frosting in an airtight container in the refrigerator. The cake can keep for 5-6 days.

Nutrition Info: Per Servings: Calories: 319 kcal, Fat: 29.2 g, Carbohydrates: 6.2 g, Protein: 7.3 g

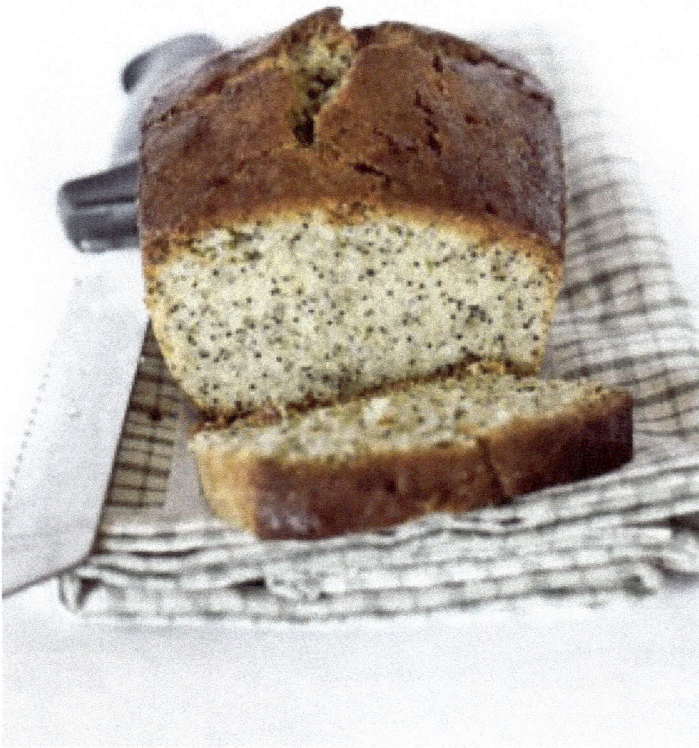

Lemon Poppy Seed Pound Cake

Servings: 8

Cooking Time: 50 Minutes

Ingredients:

- For cake (wet ingredients):
- 6 tablespoons butter, softened
- 2 large eggs, at room temperature
- 1 tablespoon lemon extract
- ½ cup erythritol
- 6 tablespoons sour cream
- 1 teaspoon vanilla extract (optional)
- For cake (dry ingredients):
- 1 ½ cups blanched almond flour
- 1 ½ tablespoons poppy seeds
- 1 teaspoon baking powder
- ¼ teaspoon sea salt
- For lemon glaze:
- 6 tablespoons powdered erythritol
- 1/8 teaspoon vanilla extract (optional)
- 2 tablespoons lemon juice

Directions:

1. Spray a small bundt pan with cooking spray.
2. Add butter and erythritol into a mixing bowl and beat with an electric hand mixer until creamy.

73

3. Add the rest of the wet ingredients and whisk well.

4. Add all dry ingredients into a bowl and stir.

5. Add dry ingredients into the bowl of wet ingredients, 1 cup at a time and mix well each time until well incorporated.

6. Spoon the batter into the bundt pan.

7. Bake in a preheated oven at 350° F for about 25-30 minutes or until dark golden brown on top. Cover the pan loosely with aluminum foil and bake for another 15-20 minutes. A toothpick when inserted in the center should come out clean when the cake is ready.

8. Cool completely. Invert onto a serving platter.

9. For glaze: Add erythritol, lemon juice and vanilla into a bowl and whisk well.

10. Pour over the cake. Spread it evenly.

11. Slice and serve.

12. Leftovers can be stored in an airtight container in the refrigerator. This can keep for a week.

Nutrition Info: Per Servings: Calories: 241.6 kcal, Fat: 22.8 g, Carbohydrates: 5.8 g, Protein: 6.8 g

Chocolate Zucchini Bundt Cake

Servings: 8

Cooking Time: 60 Minutes

Ingredients:

- For cake (dry ingredients):
- 1 ¼ cups + 2 tablespoons almond flour
- ¼ cup cacao powder
- ¼ teaspoon salt or Himalayan pink salt
- 2/3 cup powdered erythritol or Swerve
- For cake (wet ingredients)
- 3 large eggs
- 1 zucchini, pureed
- ¼ cup melted butter or ghee
- 1 teaspoon vanilla extract
- For frosting:
- 2 tablespoons virgin coconut oil
- Stevia drops to taste
- ¼ cup cacao powder

Directions:

1. Spray a small bundt pan with cooking spray.
2. Add all dry ingredients into a bowl and stir.
3. Add all wet ingredients into another bowl and whisk well.

4. Add wet ingredients into the bowl of dry ingredients and mix until well incorporated.

5. Spoon the batter into the bundt pan.

6. Bake in a preheated oven at 325° F for about 45 minutes. A toothpick when inserted in the center should come out clean when the cake is ready.

7. Cool completely. Invert onto a serving platter.

8. To make frosting: Add coconut oil and cacao powder into a small pan. Place the pan over low heat. Stir until well combined. Turn off the heat. Add stevia and stir.

9. Spread the frosting over the cake and serve.

10. Leftovers can be stored in an airtight container in the refrigerator. This can keep for a week.

Nutrition Info: Per Servings: Calories: 238.3 kcal , Fat: 21.9 g , Carbohydrates: 10.3 g , Protein: 7.3 g

Carrot Cake With Cream Cheese Frosting

Servings: 10

Cooking Time:40 Minutes

Ingredients:

- 2 cups ground almonds
- 2 tsp baking powder
- 1 tsp ground cinnamon
- ½ tsp ground allspice
- Pinch of salt
- 1 tsp Stevia/your preferred keto sweetener
- 4 eggs
- ½ cup flaxseed oil
- ¾ cup grated carrot
- 2 tsp vanilla extract
- Frosting:
- 13 oz full fat cream cheese
- 4 oz butter, softened
- 1 tsp Stevia/your preferred keto sweetener
- ½ cup chopped walnuts

Directions:

1. Preheat the oven to 360 degrees Fahrenheit and line a cake pan with baking paper
2. Toss together the ground almonds, baking powder, cinnamon, allspice, salt and sweetener in a large bowl

3. In a smaller bowl, whisk together the eggs, oil, carrot and vanilla

4. Pour the wet ingredients into the dry ingredients and stir to combine

5. Pour the batter into your prepared cake pan and place it into the preheated oven to bake for about 2minutes or until the center bounces back when gently pressed

6. Leave the cake to cool completely before frosting with cream cheese frosting

7. To make the cream cheese frosting: beat together the cream cheese, butter and sweetener until thick and creamy. Spread the frosting over the cooled cake

8. Sprinkle the chopped walnuts over the frosted cake

9. Slice and serve!

Nutrition Info: Calories: 439;Fat: 40 grams ;Protein: 13 grams ;Total carbs: grams ;Net carbs: 7 grams

Vanilla Berry Mug Cake

Servings: 1

Cooking Time: 1 Minute

Ingredients:

- 1 tbsp butter melted
- 2 tbsp cream cheese full fat
- 2 tbsp coconut flour
- 1 tbsp granulated swerve
- 1 tsp vanilla essence
- 1/4 tsp baking powder
- 1 egg medium
- 6 frozen raspberries

Directions:

1. Beat butter with cream cheese in a mug.
2. Heat this mixture in the microwave for seconds on High temperature.
3. Stir in coconut flour, baking powder, sweetener, and vanilla.
4. Mix well and whisk in the egg.
5. Once smooth, top the batter with 6 berries.
6. Cook the batter for 1 minute and 20 seconds on high temperature in the microwave.
7. Serve.

Nutrition Info: Per Servings: Calories 307 Total Fat 29 g
Saturated Fat 14g Cholesterol 111 mg Total Carbs 7 g Sugar 1 g
Fiber 3 g Sodium 122 mg Potassium 7mg Protein 6 g

Coffee Cake

Servings: 12

Cooking Time: 50 Minutes

Ingredients:

- For the cake:
- 2/3 cup coconut flour
- 1 1/4 cup monk fruit sweetener, granulated
- 2/3 cup coconut oil, softened
- 1 tsp. baking soda
- 9 large eggs
- 1/2 tsp. ground cinnamon
- 2 tsp. vanilla extract, sugar-free
- 3/4 tsp. xanthan gum
- 1/2 tsp. salt
- 2 tsp. cream of tartar
- For the topping:
- 3 tbsp. coconut flour
- 1/4 cup monk fruit sweetener, granulated
- 1 cup coconut, shredded
- 5 tbsp. coconut oil, melted
- 1 1/4 tsp. ground cinnamon

Directions:

1. Set your stove to the temperature of 350° Fahrenheit. Use butter to liberally lubricate a 9-inch square pan.

2. In a big dish, cream the eggs with an electrical beater. Add the coconut oil and vanilla extract mixing thoroughly.

3. In a separate dish, whisk the sweetener and coconut flour and blend until there are no lumps in the batter.

4. Add in the cinnamon, cream of tartar, xanthan gum and salt until incorporated.

5. Combine slowly all of the ingredients with an electrical beater until the dough forms.

6. Distribute the batter to the prepped cake pan and heat in the stove for 35 minutes.In an additional dish, whisk the sweetener and coconut with an electrical beater until mixed together. Then stir in the coconut oil, cinnamon, and coconut flour until crumbly.

7. Pull the cake out of the stove and move to the counter for 30 minutes to cool in the pan.Apply the crumble topping and slice before serving.

8. Tricks and Tips:

9. Another tip to not have the cake stick to the pan is to brush 2 teaspoons of coconut oil that has been melted along inside of the pan. Put in the freezer until you are ready to bake.

10. Take note that this recipe is a nut and dairy free, so feel free to enjoy this recipe with your morning coffee!

Nutrition Info: 5.5 grams ;Net Carbs: 1.7 grams ;Fat: 22.9 grams ;Calories: 320

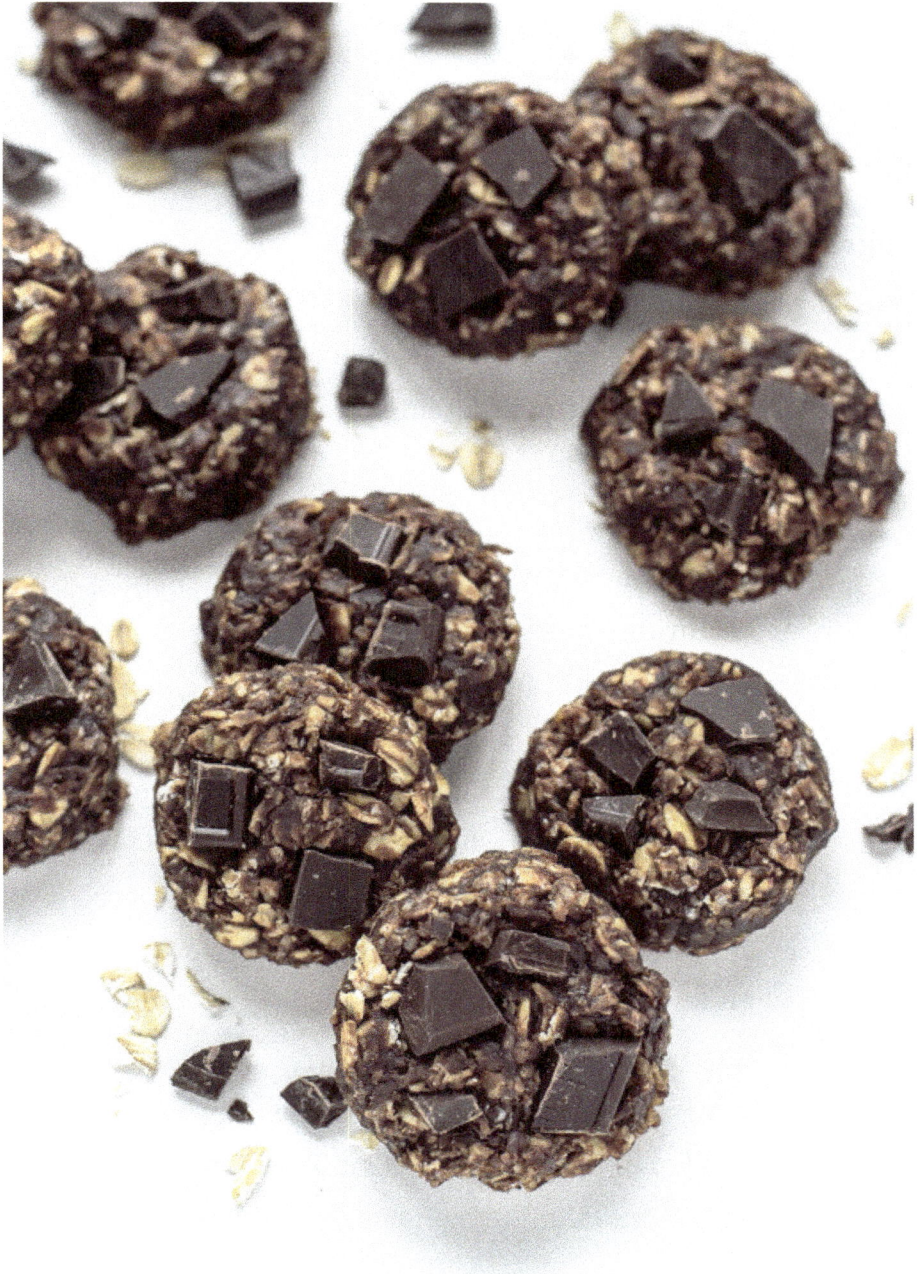

Homemade Keto Bars

Servings: 4

Cooking Time: 20 Minutes

Ingredients:

- 3/4 cup raw coconut meat
- 1/3 cup sugar free bakers' chocolate
- 2 tsp unflavoured protein powder
- 2.25 tbsp butter
- 1.5 tbsp water
- 3/4 tbsp heavy whipping cream
- Erythritol, to taste
- 35 drops liquid stevia

Directions:

1. Put all the bar ingredients in a food processor.
2. Pulse the processor to blend the ingredients well.
3. Divide this mixture into the bar molds.
4. Bake them for 20 minutes at 250 degrees F.
5. Allow them to cool.
6. Serve.

Nutrition Info: Per Servings: Calories 316 Total Fat 30.9 g Saturated Fat 8.1 g Cholesterol 0 mg Total Carbs 8.3 g Sugar 1.8 g Fiber 3.8 g Sodium 8 mg Potassium 8mg Protein 6.4 g

Protein Bar

Servings: 16

Cooking Time: 1 Hour And 5 Minutes

Ingredients:

- 4 tablespoons chocolate chips, sugar-free
- ½ teaspoon pink salt
- 1 teaspoon monk fruit
- 2 scoops vanilla protein
- 1 cup of almond butter
- 4 tablespoons coconut oil, melted

Directions:

1. Place all the ingredients in a bowl, stir well until mixed and add to a baking dish.
2. Spread the mixture evenly and place in freezer for 1 hour or more until firm.
3. Cut into bars and serve.

Nutrition Info: Calories: 280 Cal, Carbs: 8 g, Fat: 2g, Protein: 11 g, Fiber: 3 g.

Pumpkin Bars

Servings: 16

Cooking Time: 28 Minutes

Ingredients:

- 2 eggs
- 1 ½ tsp pumpkin pie spice
- ½ tsp baking soda
- 1 tsp baking powder
- ¼ cup coconut flour
- 8 oz pumpkin puree
- ½ cup coconut oil, melted
- 13 cup Swerve
- Pinch of salt

Directions:

1. Preheat the oven to 350 F 0 C.
2. Spray 9*9 inch baking pan with cooking spray and set aside.
3. In a bowl, beat eggs, sweetener, coconut oil, pumpkin pie spice, and pumpkin puree until well combined.
4. In another bowl, mix together coconut flour, baking soda, baking powder, and salt.
5. Add coconut flour mixture to the egg mixture and mix well.

6. Pour bar mixture into the prepared baking pan and spread evenly.

7. Bake in preheated oven for 28 minutes.

8. Allow to cool completely then slice and serve.

Nutrition Info: Per Servings: Net Carbs: 1.1g; Calories: 73; Total Fat: 7.5g; Saturated Fat: 6.1g Protein: 0.; Carbs: 1.6g; Fiber: 0.5g; Sugar: 0.5g; Fat 90% Protein 4% Carbs 6%

Keto Lemon Bars

Servings: 16

Cooking Time: 45 Minutes

Ingredients:

- 1 cup butter, melted
- 2 cups powdered erythritol, divided
- 6 large eggs
- 3 ½ cups almond flour, divided
- Zest of 2 lemons, grated
- Juice of 4 lemons + juice from the 2 lemons from which zest has been removed
- ¼ teaspoon salt
- To garnish:
- 4-5 thin lemon slices
- Erythritol, to sprinkle

Directions:

1. Add butter, a pinch of salt, ½ cup erythritol and 2 cups almond flour into a bowl and mix until crumbly.
2. Line a large baking dish (9 x 13) or use smaller baking dishes, with parchment paper.
3. Transfer the almond flour mixture into the baking dish. Press it well onto the bottom of the dish.

4. Bake in a preheated oven at 350° F for about 20-25 minutes or until light brown. Remove from the oven and set aside to cool for a while.

5. Add lemon zest, pinch of salt, eggs, lemon juice remaining erythritol and almond flour into a mixing bowl and mix until well combined.

6. Spoon the mixture over the crust.

7. Bake in a preheated oven at 350° F for about 20-25 minutes or until set.

8. Remove from the oven and let it cool completely.

9. Garnish with lemon slices. Dust with erythritol and serve.

10. Leftovers can be stored in an airtight container in the refrigerator. These can keep for 4 – 5 days.

Nutrition Info: Per Servings: Calories: 248.5 kcal, Fat: 23.9 g, Carbohydrates: 4.6 g, Protein: 7 g

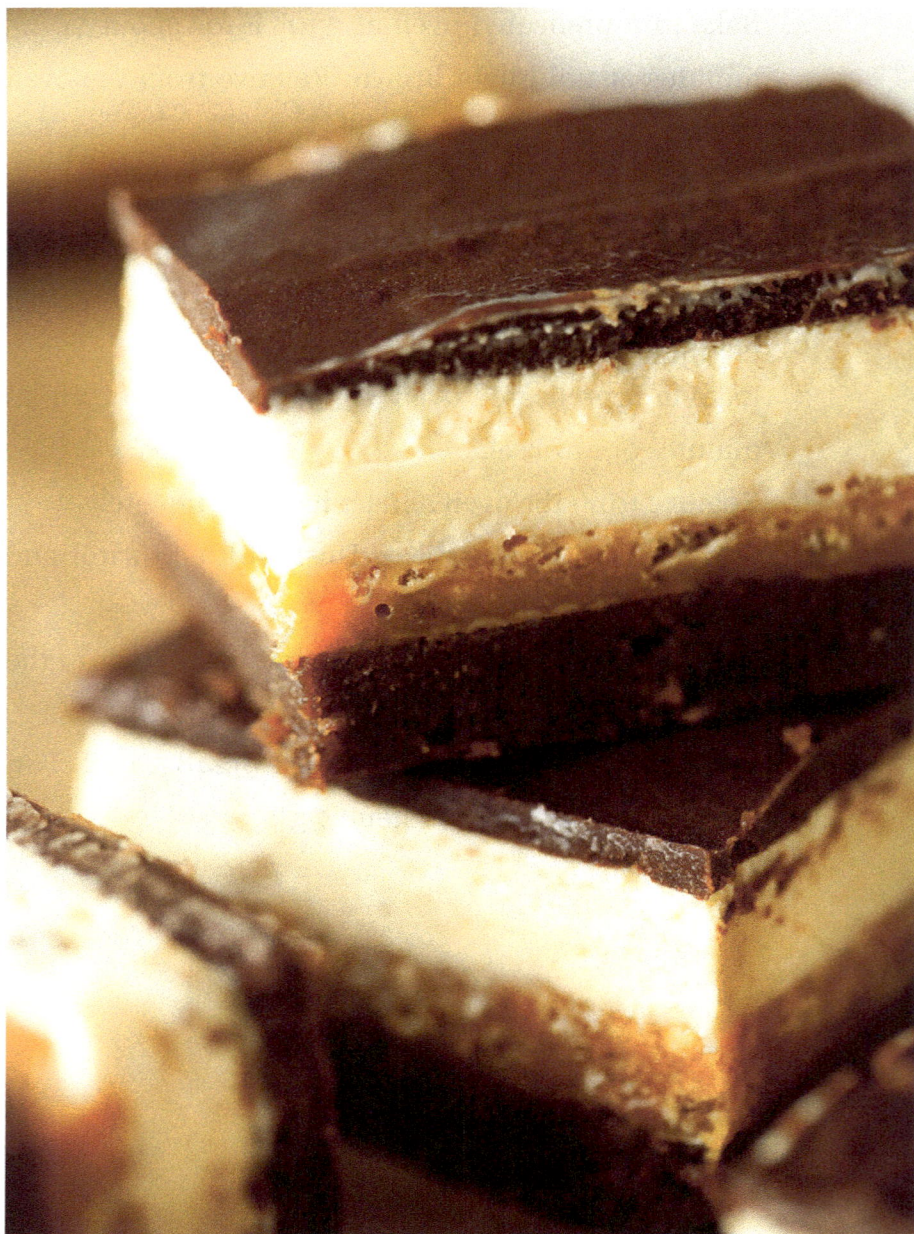

Caramel Bars

Servings: 8

Cooking Time: 40 Minutes

Ingredients:

- For the Cracker Base
- 1 cup almond flour
- 1/4 teaspoon salt
- 1/4 teaspoon baking powder
- 1 egg
- 2 tablespoons grass-fed salted butter, melted
- Caramel Sauce
- 1/2 cup Swerve
- 1/2 cup butter
- 1/2 cup heavy cream
- 1 teaspoon caramel extract
- 1/2 teaspoon vanilla essence
- 1/4 teaspoon salt
- Toppings:
- 2 cups lily's chocolate chips
- 1 cup pecans, chopped
- 1 cup coconut, shredded

Directions:

1. Crackers:
2. Let your oven preheat at 300 degrees F.

3. Combine baking powder, salt and almond flour in a suitable bowl.
4. Beat the butter in the egg until well combined.
5. Pour this butter mixture into the flour mixture and stir well to combine.
6. Place the dough on the working surface layered with parchment paper.
7. Cut the dough into a rectangle then cover it with a parchment paper.
8. Now spread it using a rolling pin into 1/inch thick dough sheet.
9. Transfer it to the baking pan and bake for 35 minutes in the preheated oven.
10. Increase the temperature of the oven to 375 degrees F.
11. Caramel sauce:
12. Put butter in a saucepan and melt it while mixing in swerve.
13. After boiling it for 7 minutes with stirring turn off the heat.
14. Stir in vanilla, cream and caramel extracts.
15. Once combined spread the sauce over the baked crackers base.
16. Drizzle chocolate chips, coconut, and pecans over it.
17. Bake for another 5 mins at the same temperature.
18. Remove it from the pan and allow it to cool and set.
19. Slice to serve.

20. Enjoy.

Nutrition Info: Calories 358 ;Total Fat 35.2 g ;Saturated Fat 15.2 g ;Cholesterol 69 mg ;Sodium 178 mg ;Total Carbs 7.4 g ;Sugar 1.1 g ;Fiber 3.5 g ;Protein 5.5 g

Chocó Chip Bars

Servings: 24

Cooking Time: 35 Minutes

Ingredients:

- 1 cup walnuts, chopped
- 1 ½ tsp baking powder
- 1 cup unsweetened chocolate chips
- 1 cup almond flour
- ¼ cup coconut flour
- 1 ½ tsp vanilla
- 5 eggs
- ½ cup butter
- 8 oz cream cheese
- 2 cups erythritol
- Pinch of salt

Directions:

1. 350 F 0 C should be the target when preheating oven.
2. Line cookie sheet with parchment paper and set aside.
3. Beat together butter, sweetener, vanilla, and cream cheese until smooth.
4. Add eggs and beat until well combined.
5. Add remaining ingredients and stir gently to combine.
6. The mixture should be transferred to the prepared cookie sheet and spread evenly.

7. Bake in preheated oven for 35 minutes.

8. Remove from oven and allow to cool completely.

9. Slice and serve.

Nutrition Info: Per Servings: Net Carbs: 2.6g; Calories: 207 Total Fat: 18.8 g; Saturated Fat: 8.5g Protein: 5.5g; Carbs: 4.8g; Fiber: 2.2g; Sugar: 0.4g; Fat 83% Protein 11% Carbs 6%

Gooey Lemon/lime Bars

Servings: 12

Cooking Time:40 Minutes

Ingredients:

- Base:
- 1 cup ground almonds
- ½ cup coconut flour
- 1 tsp Stevia/your preferred keto sweetener
- 3 oz butter, melted
- 1 egg
- 1 pinch salt
- 1 tsp baking powder
- Filling:
- Juice and zest of 3 lemons
- Juice and zest of 3 limes
- 4 eggs
- 2 tsp cornstarch dissolved in 2 Tbsp water
- 1 tsp Stevia/your preferred keto sweetener

Directions:

1. Preheat the oven to 360 degrees Fahrenheit and line a brownie pan with baking paper
2. Place all of the base ingredients into a food processor and pulse until everything comes together to form a wet, sand-like consistency

3. Press the base into the prepared pan and place into the oven to bake for 10 minutes while you prep the filling

4. Place all of the filling ingredients into the food processor (don't worry about cleaning it after making the base) and blitz until super smooth

5. Pour the filling into the pre-baked base and pop it back into the oven for about 1minutes or until just set but still a little soft and gooey

6. Leave to cool completely before slicing into bars

Nutrition Info: Calories: 156;Fat: 12 grams ;Protein: 5 grams ;Total carbs: 8 grams ;Net carbs: 4 grams

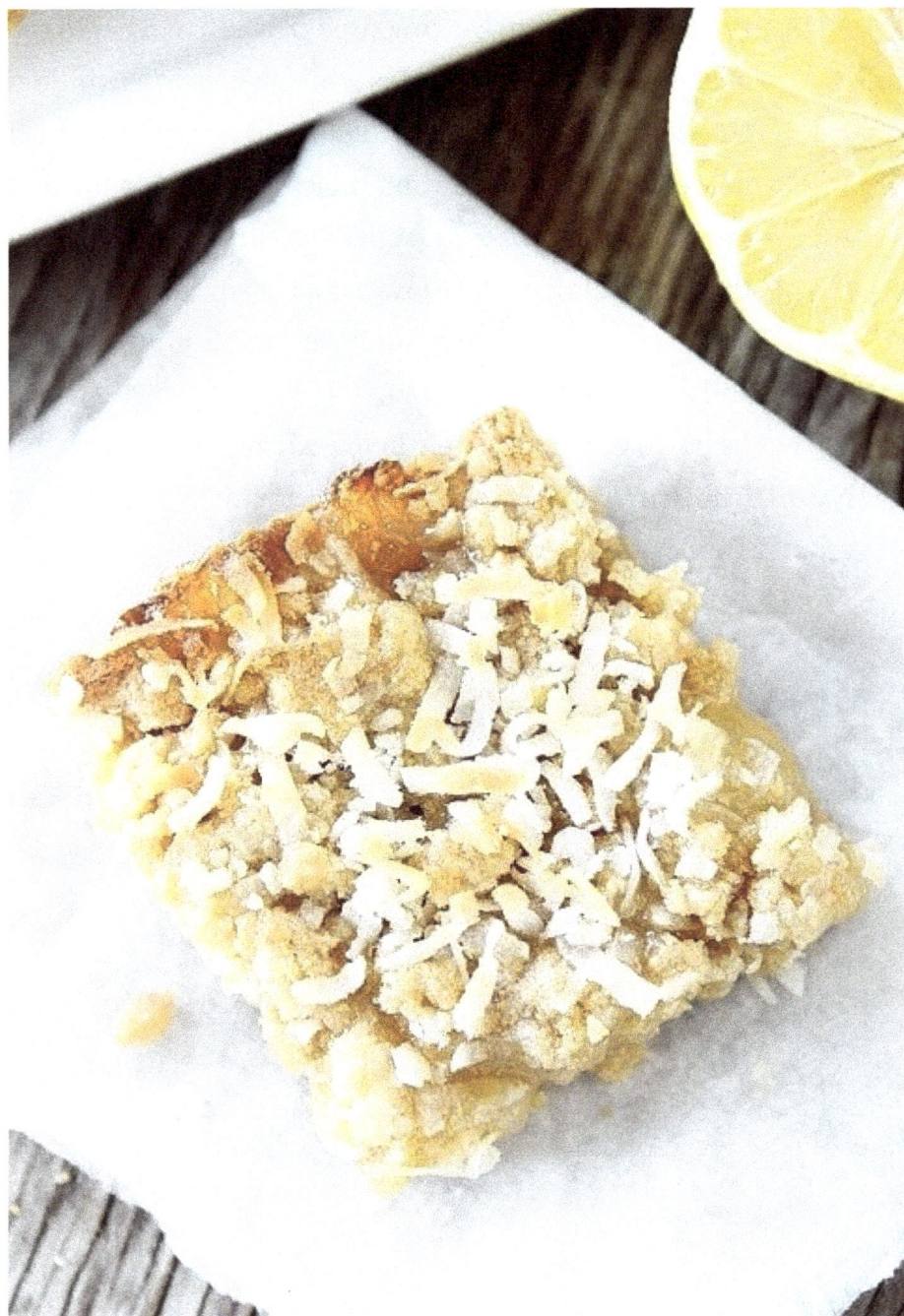

Coconut Lemon Bars

Servings: 24

Cooking Time: 42 Minutes

Ingredients:

- 4 eggs
- 1 tbsp coconut flour
- 34 cup Swerve
- 12 tsp baking powder
- 13 cup fresh lemon juice
- For crust:
- 14 cup Swerve
- 2 14 cups almond flour
- 12 cup coconut oil, melted

Directions:

1. Preheat the oven to 350 F 0 C.
2. Spray a baking dish with cooking spray and set aside.
3. In a small bowl, mix together 14 cup swerve and almond flour.
4. Add melted coconut oil and mix until it forms into a dough.
5. Transfer dough into the prepared pan and spread evenly.
6. Bake for 15 minutes.

7. For the filling: Add eggs, coconut flour, baking powder, lemon juice, and swerve into the blender and blend for 10 seconds.

8. Pour blended mixture on top of baked crust and spread well.

9. Bake for 25 minutes.

10. Remove from oven and set aside to cool completely.

11. Slice and serve.

Nutrition Info: Per Servings: Net Carbs: 1.5g; Calories: 113; Total Fat: 10.6g; Saturated Fat: 4.6g Protein: 3.3g; Carbs: 2.8g; Fiber: 1.3g; Sugar: 0.5g; Fat 84% Protein 11% Carbs 5%

Nut Bars

Servings: 10

Cooking Time: 1 Hour And 10 Minutes

Ingredients:

- ½ cup pumpkin seeds
- ½ cup sunflower seeds
- 1 tablespoon chia seeds
- 1/4 teaspoon salt
- 1/3 cup Fiber Syrup
- 1 teaspoon vanilla extract, unsweetened
- ½ cup shredded coconut, unsweetened
- 3 tablespoons almond butter
- 2 tablespoons coconut oil
- ½ cup almonds, sliced
- ½ cup walnuts, chopped

Directions:

1. Take an 8-inch baking dish, line with parchment paper, then grease with oil and set aside until required.
2. Place vanilla, fiber syrup, butter and oil in a heatproof bowl and microwave for 30 seconds or more until melted.
3. Stir well, then add remaining ingredients and stir thoroughly until combined.

4. Spoon the mixture into baking dish, press and spread evenly and place into the freezer for 1 hour or until firm.

5. Slice and serve.

Nutrition Info: Calories: 2 Cal, Carbs: 15 g, Fat: 22 g, Protein: 7 g, Fiber: 11 g.

Chocolate Bars

Servings: 12

Cooking Time: 5 Minutes

Ingredients:

- 6 ounces cocoa butter or 4 tablespoons coconut oil
- ¾ cup powdered erythritol
- ½ teaspoon liquid sunflower lecithin
- 2 teaspoons vanilla extract
- 5 ounces unsweetened baking chocolate
- 4 tablespoons inulin
- ¼ teaspoon sea salt

Directions:

1. Add chocolate and cocoa butter into a heatproof bowl.
2. Place the bowl in a double boiler. Stir occasionally until the mixture melts.
3. Add erythritol, 2 tablespoons at a time and mix well each time. Add inulin, a tablespoon at a time and mix well each time. When the mixture is smooth and well incorporated, turn off the heat.
4. Add vanilla and mix well.
5. Spoon into 12 chocolate molds. Cool completely.
6. Chill until firm. Remove from mold and serve.
7. Leftovers can be stored in an airtight container in the refrigerator. These can keep for 4 – 5 days.

Nutrition Info: Per Servings: Calories: 177.75 kcal, Fat: 19 g, Carbohydrates: 4.25 g, Protein: 1.4 g

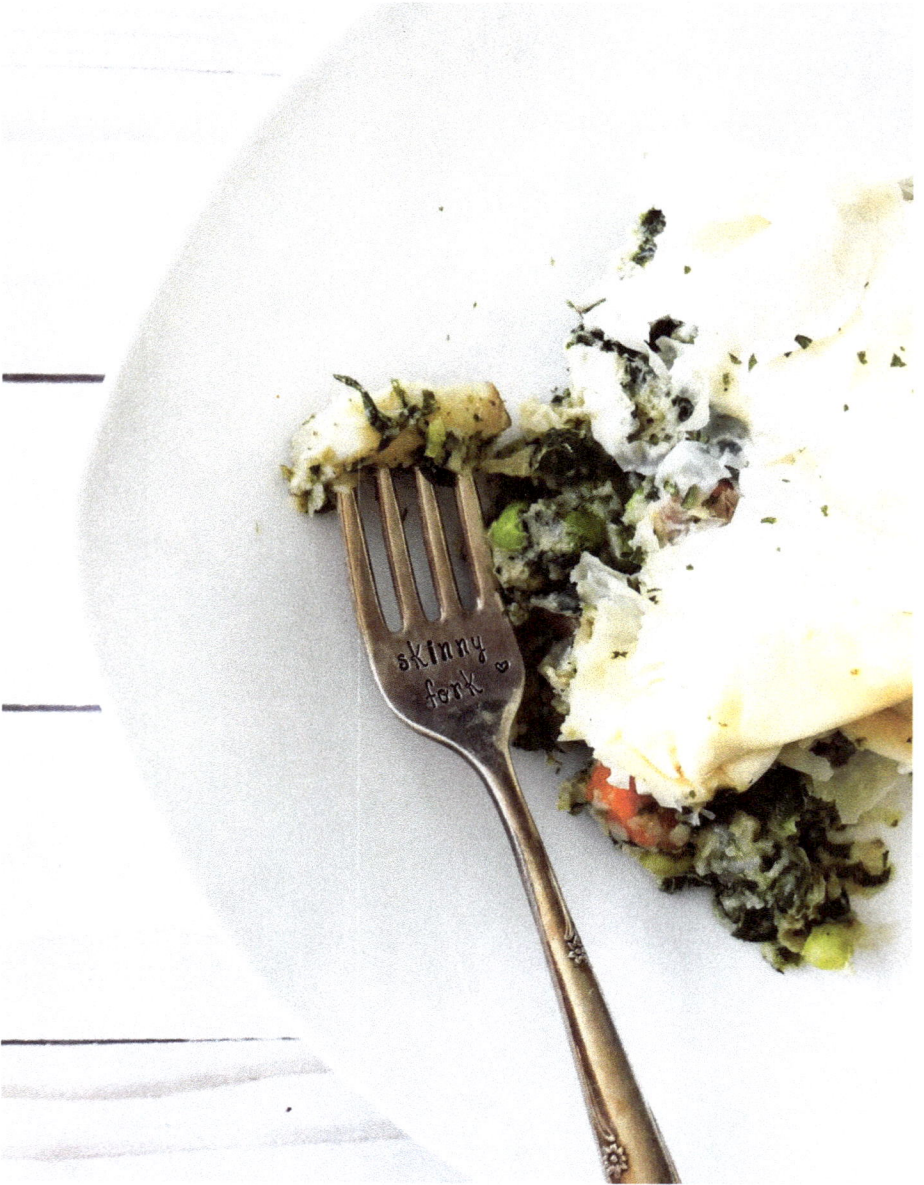

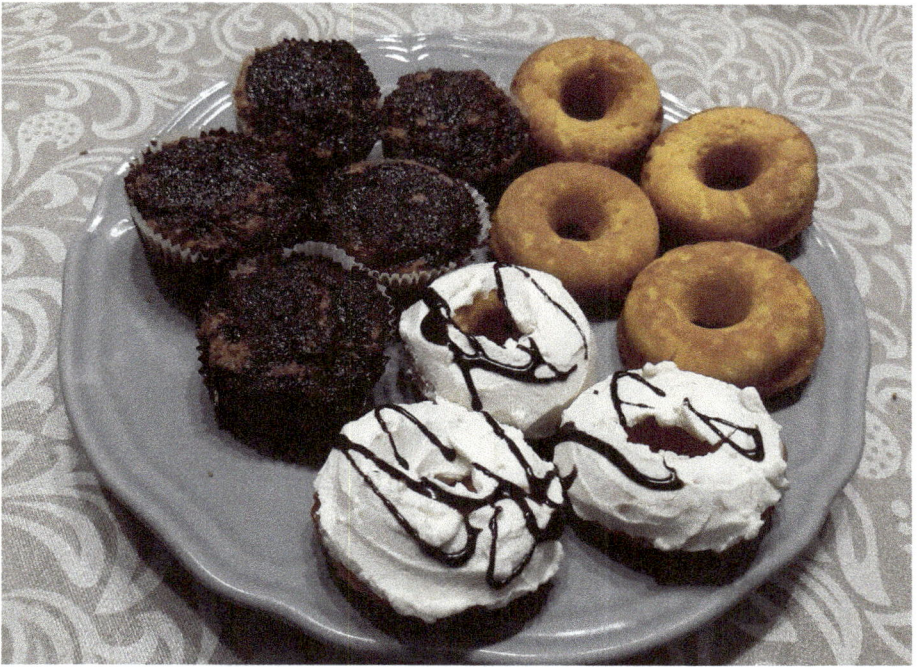

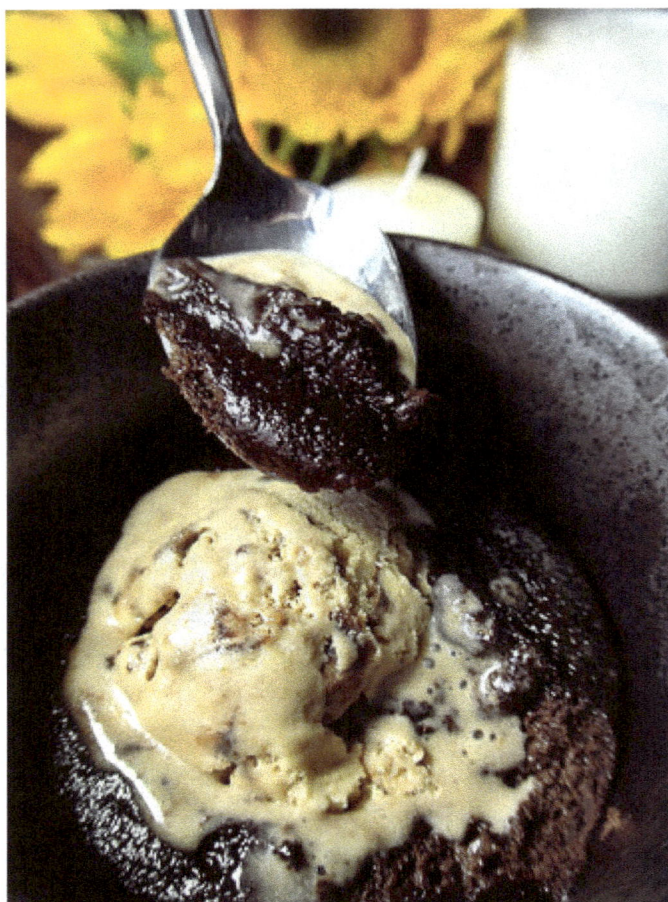

www.ingramcontent.com/pod-product-compliance
Lightning Source LLC
Chambersburg PA
CBHW062119040426
42336CB00041B/1957